DIGITAL SIGNAL
AND IMAGE
PROCESSING
IN JAGIELLONIAN
POSITRON EMISSION
TOMOGRAPHY

LECH RACZYŃSKI

DIGITAL SIGNAL AND IMAGE PROCESSING IN JAGIELLONIAN POSITRON EMISSION TOMOGRAPHY

Jagiellonian
University
Press

The publication of this volume was financed by the National Centre for Nuclear Research

REVIEW
Prof. dr hab. Jerzy Smyrski

COVER DESIGN
Mateusz Otręba

ISBN 978-83-233-5015-6
ISBN 978-83-233-7249-3 (e-book)

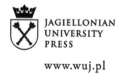

JAGIELLONIAN
UNIVERSITY
PRESS

www.wuj.pl

Jagiellonian University Press
Editorial Offices: Michalowskiego 9/2, 31-126 Kraków
Phone: +48 12 663 23 80, Fax: +48 12 663 23 83
Distribution: Phone: +48 12 631 01 97, Fax: +48 12 631 01 98
Cell Phone: +48 506 006 674, e-mail: sprzedaz@wuj.pl
Bank: PEKAO SA, IBAN PL 80 1240 4722 1111 0000 4856 3325

Habilitation thesis prepared at the Department of Complex Systems in the National Centre for Nuclear Research, submitted to the National Centre for Nuclear Research, for the postdoctoral lecture qualification.

Acknowledgements

Accomplishing of experiments and simulations presented in this dissertation was possible only due to the joined effort of many colleagues from the J-PET collaboration whom I had the luck to work with. First of all, I would like to thank Professor Wojciech Wiślicki, director of the Department of Complex Systems in National Centre for Nuclear Research (my workplace) and Professor Paweł Moskal, inventor of the J-PET tomograph and founder of the J-PET collaboration.

I am profoundly grateful to Professor Wojciech Wiślicki for inviting me to the J-PET sub-group that he founded in our institute in 2012. I could always count on his help and advices when I was facing difficult scienctific and administrative problems. I am greatly indebted to Professor Paweł Moskal for the extremely skilful coordination of the J-PET project. I admire him for his inexhaustible enthusiasm and his dedication to the project. By the side of Professor Wojciech Wiślicki and Professor Paweł Moskal, I have learned that you can love the work you do.

I wish also to express my thanks to all colleagues from the J-PET collaboration for their help and friendliness. I was pleased to work together with many kind and talented people. In particular, I am very grateful to Doctor Wojciech Krzemień and Doctor Konrad Klimaszewski for fruitful discussions and friendly atmosphere during our numerous meetings. I wish also to express my thanks to Przemysław Kopka and Paweł Kowalski for providing numercial simulations of the J-PET detector.

Preparation of this work would not be possible without support and involvement of my family. I am deeply indebted to my wife Małgorzata, my daughter Agata, my parents Anna and Andrzej, and my late aunt Zofia for believing in me and encouraging me throughout this journey. Especially, I would like to thank and dedicate this work to my wife Małgorzata for creating great conditions for my scientific work in our home and teaching me what true sacrifice means.

Contents

Abbreviations

AFOV	axial field of view
BMU	best matching unit
BPF	back-projection filter
BPTV	back-projection total variation
BV	background variability
cdf	cumulative distribution function
CRC	contrast recovery coefficient
CRT	coincidence resolving time
CS	compressive sensing
DOI	depth-of-interaction
FBP	filtered back-projection
F-FDG	fludeoxy-D-glucose
FOV	field of view
FPGA	field-programmable gate array
FWHM	full width at half-maximum
GATE	Geant4 application for tomographic emission
J-PET	Jagiellonian PET
LDA	linear discriminant analysis
LM	list-mode
LOR	line of response
LSO	lutetium oxyorthosilicate
MC	monte carlo

MCP	microchannel plates photomultiplier
MLEM	maximum likelihood expectation maximization
MVN	multivariate normal distribution
NEMA	national electrical manufacturers association
PCA	principal component analysis
pdf	probability density function
PET	positron emission tomography
PM	photomultiplier
PMT	photomultiplier tube
PPV	positive predictive value
PSF	point spread function
RMSE	root mean square error
ROI	region of interest
SiPM	silicon photomultiplier
SNR	signal to noise ratio
SOM	self-organizing map
TDC	time-to-digital converter
TOF	time of flight
TPR	true positive rate
TR	Tikhonov regularization
TV	total variation

Preface

Results constituting the basis for this dissertation have been published in seven articles [1–7] and presented at eight conferences. The research has been realized at the Jagiellonian University by means of the Jagiellonian PET scanner. Ideas of proposed signal and image processing have been positively judged and approved for application by the Jagiellonian PET collaboration.

1. Introduction

Positron Emission Tomography (PET) is at present one of the most technologically advanced diagnostic methods for non-invasive imaging in medicine [8,9]. It plays a unique role both in medical diagnostics and in monitoring effects of therapy, in particular in oncology, cardiology, neurology and psychiatry. In PET measurement the patient is injected with radiotracer, containing a large number of metastable atoms of positron emitting radionuclide. Since the rate of assimilation of radiopharmaceuticals depends on the type of the tissues, sections of the diseased cells can be identified with high accuracy, even if they are not yet detectable via morphological changes. Therefore, PET is extremely effective in locating and diagnosing cancer metastases.

As the result of positron annihilation, two photons travelling off with nearly opposite directions are produced. The detection system is usually arranged in layers forming a ring around the diagnosed patient. In the basic PET measurement scheme, the information about the single event of positron annihilation is collected in the form of a line joining the detected locations that passes directly through the point of annihilation, i.e. the Line-of-Response (LOR). The set of registered LORs forms the basis for PET image reconstruction. New generation of PET scanners utilizes not only information about the LORs but also takes advantage of the measurement of the time difference between the arrival of the two photons at the detectors, referred to as the Time-Of-Flight (TOF) difference [10]. State-of-the-art TOF-PET scanners use scintillation crystals and operate at a time resolution, defined hereafter as the coincidence resolving time (CRT), of the order of $300-400$ ps [11, 12]. The fundamental improvement brought by TOF is an increase in signal-to-noise ratio (SNR); in the first approximation the SNR improvement due to TOF application is inversely proportional to the square root of the CRT [13]. For example, if a time resolution of 400 ps is applied, this yields, for a patient of about 40 cm average transaxial size, an SNR about three times better than for non TOF information measurement. The time resolution achievable with the scintillator detectors is limited by the optical and electronic time spread caused by the detector components, and by the time distribution of photons contributing to the formation of electric signals. A detailed elaboration of the lower bound for time resolution has been published for most kinds of available crystal scintillators in [14]. The modern technology of lutetium oxyorthosilicate (LSO) crystals is particularly promising, as it shows an excellent timing resolution. Studies using small LSO crystals indicate the timing limit at the level of about 100 ps [15]. Recent theoretical studies indicate that there are no physical barriers to reaching the resolution of about 10 ps in the future [16].

In this context, it is worth to mention that the Jagiellonian PET (J-PET) Collaboration developed a novel whole-body PET scanner based on plastic scintillators [17–20]. Plastic scintillators are characterized by superior timing properties compared to scintillator crystals. The TOF resolution achievable with plastic scintillators may be even better than 100 ps for a large detector, even in the scale of one meter [19], and plastic scintillators can be produced easily in variety of shapes and dimensions. Detectors based on plastic scintillators are commonly used in nuclear and particle physics experiments, however, due to negligible probability of photo-electric effect, their potential for registration of low energy photon, in the range of 511 keV, was so far not explored except for few publications concentrated on the light propagation studies or callibration methods [21, 22].

The operational principles of the J-PET detector are similar to conventional scanners, except that the highly accurate time information is of paramount importance. State-of-the-art crystal based scanners use TOF to improve the quality of the reconstructed image, but they can as well operate in basic scheme, relying only on information from LORs. In case of the J-PET, as it will be discussed in detail in the next chapters, however, the accurate time information is essential to perform a signal reconstruction. Therefore, the J-PET tomograph demands a preparation of novel methods at each step of data processing. The goal of the work presented in this dissertation is a development of the signal and image processing methods taking into account the uniqueness of the J-PET detector. Due to the dissimilarity from the conventional PET scanners, a majority of the methods presented in this work are innovative solutions in digital data processing in tomography.

This dissertation is organized into seven chapters. After this introduction the basics of PET physics and measurement techniques will be elucidated and the main aspects of the data processing in the Jagiellonian PET will be presented and discussed. Further, in the third chapter, a short overview of the state-of-the-art algorithms that contributed to the development of new concepts of signal processing and image reconstruction will be given. That chapter precedes a presentation of the subsequent steps of the developed data processing methods that will be described in chapters four and five. The fourth chapter presents an original approach to signal recovery and reconstruction, denoted in this work with low-level signal processing, dedicated to the TOF-PET scanners. The fifth chapter discusses high-level image processing. In order to perform image reconstruction for the J-PET detector, a specific statistical model that describes the probability density function of annihilation position, including time measurement errors, will be introduced. A detailed descriptions of the simulation and experimental studies and the comparison results are given in the sixth chapter. The conclusions and directions for future work are presented in chapter seven. The dissertation is supplied with appendices containing derivation of math proofs that constitute the main individual contribution to the digital signal and image processing in tomography.

2. Positron Emission Tomography

The first demonstration of PET technique for medical imaging use was given in early 1950s by Brownell and Burnham. This was an inspiration for the concept of emission tomography used to visualize functional processes in the body in the late 1950s. The first 3-dimensional PET detector, called PC-1, was developed at the Massachusetts General Hospital and completed in 1969. This PET device comprised two planar opposed arrays of crystal scintillators [23]. In 1973 Robertson and his co-workers built the first ring PET scanner, which consisted of 32 detectors [24]. The cylindrical array of detectors has soon become the prototype of the current shape of PET [25].

The fundamental requirement that comes together with the development of the PET technology was to create radiopharmaceutical tracers that could be administered safely to the patient's body. Currently, the most important radiopharmaceutical in PET examinations is fludeoxy-D-glucose (^{18}F-FDG) [26]. ^{18}F-FDG is an analog of glucose used for cellular metabolism having the hydroxyl group replaced by radionuclide ^{18}F. Radionuclide ^{18}F is produced in a cyclotron and has a relatively long half-life, about 110 min, that allows its supply to remote places. Similarly as glucose, ^{18}F-FDG is absorbed by brain or kidney cells, and what is most important, by the cancer cells presenting abnormally high metabolism in comparison to the healthy organs. Therefore, PET imaging presents the distribution of glucose consumption by the cells and an overall cellular activity in the patient body.

Radionuclides are unstable due to the unsuitable composition of neutrons and protons and, therefore, decay by emission of radiation. When a radionuclide is proton rich, as in the case of ^{18}F, it decays by the emission of a positron (β^+) along with a neutrino (v):

$$^{1}_{1}\text{p}^+ \rightarrow {}^{1}_{0}\text{n} + {}^{0}_{1}\beta^+ + v. \tag{2.1}$$

For instance, the scheme for positron decay from ^{18}F is:

$$^{18}_{9}\text{F} \rightarrow {}^{18}_{8}\text{O} + {}^{0}_{1}\beta^+ + v. \tag{2.2}$$

The stability of radionuclide is achieved by converting a proton ($_1^1\mathrm{p}^+$) in the nucleus to a neutron ($_0^1\mathrm{n}$). Since a daughter nucleus is one atomic number smaller than a parent nucleus, one of the orbital electrons has to be ejected from the atom. As both an electron and β^+ are emitted in the decay described in Eq. (2.1), the right-hand side of this formula has to be at least two electron mass more than the left-hand side, i.e., 2×511 keV $= 1022$ keV. The energy beyond 1022 keV is shared as kinetic energy by β^+ and a neutrino.

After emission from the nucleus, β^+ particle loses kinetic energy by interactions with the surrounding matter. The range of positron depends on many parameters such as the energy, charge as well as the density of the matter it passes through. Therefore an empirical measurements are usually provided to estimate the mean positron range in a given material [27]. When a kinetic energy of β^+ particle approaches zero, positron combines with an electron and both annihilate as a result of matter-antimatter interaction. The positron-electron annihilation may proceed directly or via formation of the intermediate positron-electron bound state referred to as positronium. Positronium is a non-nuclear form composed of the positron and electron that revolve around their combined centre of mass. Positronium formation occurs with a high probability in gases and metals, while in human tissue or water a direct annihilation of the electron and the β^+ particle is more likely, i.e., in about two-third of all cases. As a result of matter-antimatter annihilation electromagnetic radiation is given off. The most probable form that this radiation takes is of two γ photons of 511 keV emitted back-to-back. Measurement of the two opposite γ photons in coincidence by a pair of detectors is the basis of PET. However, due to non-zero kinetic energies of positron and electron in the moment of annihilation, the two γ photons are not emitted exactly at 180°. This effect together with the non-zero range of the β^+ particle before annihilation, gives a fundamental lower limit of the spatial resolution of PET images.

2.1   Interaction of γ photons with matter

The electromagnetic radiation in form of 511 keV γ photons is highly penetrating. γ photons interact with matter by three main mechanisms: photoelectric effect, Compton scattering, and pair production. The relative domination of these three interaction types depends on the γ photon energy and on the absorbing material atomic number. Since in discussion of PET technology we focus on the 511 keV γ photons, only two first mechanism of interactions, i.e., photoelectric effect and Compton scattering, are considered. Pair production may be omitted, since the energy of at least 1022 keV is required to initiate this mechanism.

2.1.1 Photoelectric effect

In the photoelectric effect, a γ photon is absorbed by the atom and its energy is transferred to remove an electron from one of the atom inner shells. The difference between the initial γ photon energy, denoted hereafter as E_γ, and the binding energy of the electron in the shell is given as the kinetic energy of ejected electron [28]. The vacancy created by the electron is filled by the electron of outer orbital followed by emission of the characteristics X-ray or an Auger electron.

The rough approximation of the probability of the photoelectric effect may be given by [29]

$$\mathbb{P}_{\mathrm{pe}} = Z_{\mathrm{eff}}^5 / E_\gamma^3 \qquad (2.3)$$

where Z_{eff} is an effective atomic number of the material and energy of γ photon (E_γ) is given in keV. The dependence of the $\mathbb{P}_{\mathrm{pe}}$ on the effective atomic number for 511 keV annihilation γ photons is shown in Fig. 2.1. As seen in Fig. 2.1, the photoelectric effect in human tissue (Z_{eff} below 10) has negligible impact at energies of annihilation γ photons. However, the probability of this process increases with increasing effective atomic number of the absorber.

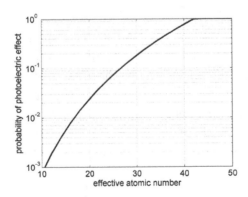

Figure 2.1.   Approximation of probability of the photoelectric effect for 511 keV γ photon.

Ahead of the facts, we would like to stress that according to the relation shown in Fig. 2.1, the photoelectric effect is the main mechanism of interaction enabling the detection of the γ photons in state-of-the-art

PET scanners; the effective atomic number of the scintillating detectors is of order of 50. This topic will be covered in detail in section 2.2.1.

2.1.2 Compton scattering

In contrast to the photoelectric effect, in the Compton scattering the γ photon interacts with an outer shell electron of the absorber material. The γ photon is not absorbed by the atom, but is scattered with reduced energy. The energy of the annihilation γ photon after the Compton scattering (E'_γ) is the specific solution of the Compton equation, where $E_\gamma = 511$ keV corresponds to the rest mass energy of the electron, and therefore [28]:

$$E'_\gamma = \frac{E_\gamma}{2 - \cos(\theta_s)} \tag{2.4}$$

where θ_s is the scattering angle. Depending on the energy E'_γ, scattered γ photon may again interact with the absorber. The Compton scattering is the main mechanism of interaction in human tissue at energies of annihilation γ photons; as shown in Fig. 2.1 for small Z_{eff} the probability of the photoelectric effect is negligible. The numerous studies of the interaction of 511 keV γ photons with tissue-equivalent material have demonstrated that in most cases, scattered photons detected during PET examinations have undergone only single scattering interaction [30].

2.1.3 Attenuation of γ radiation

Single annihilation γ photon may interact with absorber material via photoelectric effect or Compton scattering, or may pass through without any interactions. For a beam of photons it is preferred to consider the global parameter that describes the combined efficiency of all types of interactions in the absorber. This parameter is denoted as attenuation coefficient (μ_{tot}) and for γ photons with energies below 1022 keV, including annihilation γ photons, is defined as [31]

$$\mu_{\mathrm{tot}} = \mu_{\mathrm{pe}} + \mu_{\mathrm{c}} \tag{2.5}$$

where μ_{pe} is the photoelectric effect coefficient and μ_{c} is the Compton scattering coefficient. For a well-collimated beam of photons, attenuation takes the form of an exponential function with a constant value μ_{tot}, i.e.,

$$I(z) = I_0 \cdot \exp\left(-\mu_{\mathrm{tot}} \cdot z\right), \tag{2.6}$$

where I_0 stands for the initial photon beam intensity and $I(z)$ is the photon beam intensity after passing through distance z in material with attenuation coefficient μ_{tot}.

2.2 Detection of γ photons

The basis of the detection of γ photons in PET technique is the interaction of radiation with scintillation detectors. The scintillation process relies on the absorption of the γ photon and conversion of its energy into a pulse of visible light. For typical scintillators, from several to several dozen thousand of photons are emitted isotropically for a single 511 keV γ photon. The rate of emission has an exponential distribution with a constant value referred to as decay time. Depending on the emission angle, part of the light escapes from the scintillator and the rest undergoes internal reflection. Part of the light photons reach the photomultiplier (PM) attached to one or more faces of the scintillation detector. The light photons in PM are converted to an electrical signal and the integral of this signal (charge) is proportional to the energy deposited in the scintillator by γ photon.

The overall charge spectrum of 511 keV γ photons acquired by the detection system is broad and fluctuating; the photopeak that arrives from the deposition of the total energy via photoelectric effect constitutes only a small part of the spectrum. The continuous values of charge (energy) represent incomplete deposition of energy by the annihilation γ photons, e.g., due to one or more Compton scattering in the tissue. The fluctuations in the acquired spectrum arise primarily from the statistical nature of the conversion process of the deposited energy into charge. The ability of the PET system to accurately measure the deposited energy is of main importance.

2.2.1 Scintillation detectors

As gas and liquid scintillators have low detection efficiency, PET technology is based on the solid scintillation detectors. Currently, two types of solid scintillators are considered for PET studies: inorganic crystals and organic plastics, however, all commercial PET devices use inorganic crystals. Plastic scintillators were not applied to PET technology due to their low μ_{tot} for annihilation γ photons and small effective atomic number of elements constituting the material.

Attenuation coefficient for 511 keV γ photons for the plastic scintillator BC-420 equals 0.098 cm^{-1} [32] and is about nine times smaller than for common crystals like bismuth germanate (BGO) $\mu_{tot} = 0.950$ cm^{-1} or lutetium oxyorthosilicate (LSO) $\mu_{tot} = 0.866$ cm^{-1} [33]. Consequently, for a 2 cm thick scintillator the probability that annihilation γ photons react in the detector amounts to about 0.2 for the plastic and about 0.8 for the crystal.

Plastic scintillators are composed mainly of carbon and hydrogen. The effective atomic number of the scintillator determines the mechanism of interactions of γ photons with the material. As shown in Fig. 2.1, small atomic number corresponds to small probability that annihilation γ photons transfer all their energy to the electrons in the scintillator through the photoelectric effect. Instead, γ radiation interacts with plastic scintillator predominantly via Compton scattering and may deposit maximally an energy of about 341 keV (see Eq. (2.4) for details). Therefore, the measured spectrum of energies of annihilation γ photons does not include the photopeak around 511 keV and the valuable signal is concentrated in the continuous part of the Compton region.

On the positive side, plastic scintillators have long light attenuation length in comparison to crystal scintillators. As a result, enough light photons reach PM in order to produce valuable signal when using scintillators in form of long strips. Long crystal scintillators would simply absorb all of the light photons before they arrived to PMs. Moreover, the extremely short decay time of plastic scintillator BC-420 of about 1.5 ns [32] is much better in comparison to best decay time of crystal scintillator of about 16 ns for cerium doped lanthanum bromide (LaBr$_3$:Ce) [33]. Due to high costs, hygroscopicity and relatively small efficiency for the photoelectric effect, the LaBr$_3$:Ce is not regarded as the material of choice for the PET detectors. The relative price of the LaBr$_3$:Ce crystal is about 230 times greater than that of the plastic scintillator BC-420 [32]. The unique timing properties of the BC-420 scintillators led to the development of the first prototype PET device based on plastic detectors. This idea will be introduced in section 2.3.

2.2.2   Light detection with photomultipliers

Photomultiplier tubes (PMTs) are the most commonly used photodetectors in PET. This detector is a vacuum glass tube containing a photocathode at one end, several dynodes in the middle, and an anode at the other end. Typically high voltage of about 1 kV is applied across the tube

to keep about 100 V increments between the dynodes [34]. Light photons strike the photocathode and knock out low energy electrons called
photoelectrons, from the photoemissive material via photoelectric effect.
Photoelectrons are accelerated toward the next closest dynode and the
process continues until the last dynode is reached. Typical gain of PMT
is in the range from 10^5 to 10^7 and leads to very good signal to noise
ratio. The main drawback of PMT is low quantum efficiency of about
20% [35].

2.3   Introduction of the Jagiellonian PET detector

In state-of-the-art PET scanners, the crystals are arranged in small
blocks [36]. Typically, each block is an array (e.g., 8 × 8) of small elements separated from each other with reflective material. The readout
in the block design is performed by a set of photomultipliers attached
directly to the scintillator surface. The amplitude distribution of the
electric signals in the photomultiplier's output allows to determine the
place of interaction of γ photon within the crystal with an accuracy
equivalent to the size of the smallest crystal element.

Clinical PET scanners are typically arranged in an array of rings with
a diameter of about 80 cm. These devices have a relatively small axial
field of view (AFOV) of about 20 cm, which offers limited body coverage
and low photon detection efficiency [37, 38]. Currently in order to perform a full body PET scan, multiple images at different bed positions
are acquired. The whole-body devices are equipped with a computer-
controlled moving bed, so that the patient can be positioned at different
locations along the AFOV. The total scan time depends on the patient's
body length and the effective AFOV of the scanner per bed position.
Since the sensitivity decreases toward the periphery of the scanner, the
effective AFOV is less than the actual FOV and it is necessary to overlap the bed positions in whole-body imaging. A typical overlap is about
5 cm. The time for data acquisition at each bed position in whole-body
imaging is about 5 min. Therefore, the whole examination takes about
30 minutes and often requires the person being scanned to stay still in
an uncomfortable position for the entire scan.

Few pioneering projects propose the construction of a whole-body
PET scanner so that the entire human body can be imaged at once.
These new devices would be a notable change from what is possible
with current PET scanners in terms of examination time or measurement precision. The whole-body technique would increase the effective

sensitivity, decrease the time of the examination and reduce the necessary image blur caused by the patient's or scanner's movements when the whole body has to be examined. The dynamic range of the whole-body scanners is much broader than of current tomographs with small AFOV, i.e., the radiotracers may be tracked for a longer time without temporal gaps [39]. The whole-body PET scanners would be able to detect very small metastatic tumors or track whether a therapy is hitting its intended target. Alternatively, the increased sensitivity could mean that far lower doses of radioactive tracers will be required for a scan [40].

The Explorer collaboration [41,42] has built a 200 cm long whole-body PET system that will have more than 400,000 crystals in total. The scanner consists of 36 axial block rings composed of LSO scintillators with an axial gap corresponding to one crystal pitch between adjacent rings. Each ring has 48 detector modules forming a ring of 80 cm in diameter [43]. The schematic visualisation of 3-dimensional geometry of 4 axial block rings of the Explorer scanner is shown on the left of Fig. 2.2.

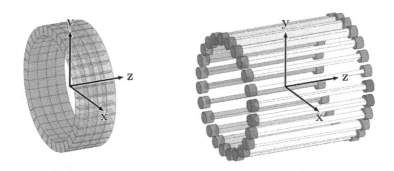

Figure 2.2. Comparison of the concepts of state-of-the-art PET scanner based on inorganic crystals (left) and the J-PET scanner (right). The figure is adapted from [44].

On the other hand, the J-PET collaboration aims at the construction of the PET scanner with a large AFOV and a superior timing resolution due to the use of fast plastic scintillators instead of inorganic crystals [17–19,45,46]. Multiple small crystal scintillators along axial coordinate (z) are replaced with a single scintillator strip in the J-PET detector. This significantly reduces the number of photomultipliers, cables and electronic boards in the PET device, therefore substantially lowering production costs. In the J-PET device the readout in single strip is provided by a pair of photomultipliers placed outside of the detection chamber, marked with small grey barrels in Fig. 2.2. This approach simplifies the combining of PET with other modalities (magnetic resonance or computed tomography) and enables extension of the AFOV without a significant increase in cost. The axial coordinate (z) of the annihilation photon interaction point in the strip is derived from the difference of the light propagation time measured with the pair of photomultipliers. The schematic visualisation of the J-PET tomograph is shown on the right of Fig. 2.2.

2.3.1   Coincidence detection of γ photons

During the PET examination, two annihilation γ photons may be emitted from anywhere within the scanner volume and the distance travelled by each of them before interaction in the detectors can be as large as the scanner diagonal. The larger the scanner FOV, the longer the maximum timing difference between the detection of two γ photons in coincidence. Using the value of speed of light, one may calculate that for a 100 cm scanner FOV a maximum timing difference of about 3 ns between the two detected signals is expected. The coincidence timing window cannot be reduced to less than that value due to the possibility of annihilation at the edge of the scanner volume. Therefore, the uncertainty of time measurement in a PET system should not be higher than the size of this time window.

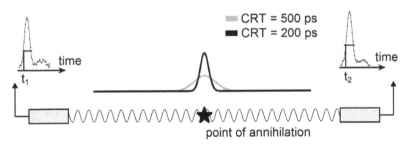

Figure 2.3. Schematic representation of detecting two γ photons in coincidence. Detection results in estimation of times t_1 and t_2 and the position of annihilation is reconstructed based on the times difference.

Figure 2.3 illustrates a schematic representation of two detectors set up to measure two γ photons emitted from a point equidistant from both detectors (marked with a black star). The times t_1 and t_2 define the signal arrival times in detectors on the left and right side, respectively.

In the simplest case, the t_1 and t_2 may be derived as the times when the registered signals cross a certain fixed voltage level. The first of the signals, i.e., the one with estimated arrival time t_1, triggers a pulse that marks the start of the coincidence window of predefined width. Measured difference between the times t_2 and t_1 depends on the time resolution of the PET system; the better the time resolution the smaller the difference of times t_2 and t_1. The estimated position of annihilation point may be estimated as:

$$\frac{c \cdot (t_2 - t_1)}{2} \tag{2.7}$$

where c is the speed of light; whereas in fact in example in Fig. 2.3, the γ photons arrived at both detectors simultaneously. The parameter that describes the time uncertainty of this measurement is called CRT. The CRT is defined as the Full Width at Half-Maximum (FWHM) of the distribution of time difference between t_2 and t_1.

As mentioned before, the minimal required time resolution of a PET system has to enable a detection of two γ photons from a single annihilation, i.e., times t_1 and t_2 need to be specified with uncertainty of at least 3 ns. In that case two detected γ photons, registered within the predefined time window, mark only a LOR between the two respective detectors. The PET systems that allow for more precise location of the position of annihilation are called time-of-flight PET (TOF-PET) scanners. The schematic visualization of the uncertainties for measurement of annihilation position in PET systems with CRT of about 500 ps and 200 ps are marked in Fig. 2.3 with grey and black Gaussian functions, respectively. The 500 ps time resolution is sufficient to localize a tumor with the size of about 7.5 cm. Reducing the CRT to 200 ps, improves the spatial resolution to 3 cm. Very good time resolution of a PET system allows to estimate the annihilation position between the two detectors by looking at the difference in arrival times of the two photons. For this purpose, an extremely fast scintillator, such as plastic BC-420, is required. It was shown recently in [19] that the physical limitation for the CRT with the J-PET system amounts to about 50 ps for the 50 cm long scintillator.

2.3.2   Time based measurement in the J-PET scanner

In classical PET scanners based on crystal scintillators, the CRT does not play a crucial role for the detection of two γ photons from single annihilation, i.e., time resolution has to be sufficient to indicate single LOR.

Therefore, conventional PET detectors can optionally use TOF information to improve the quality of reconstructed images. However, in case of
the J-PET scanner, the accurate timing is mandatory to reconstruct the
position along the strip. The schematic visualisation of reconstruction of
position along z direction for the J-PET scanner is shown on the right
of Fig. 2.4.

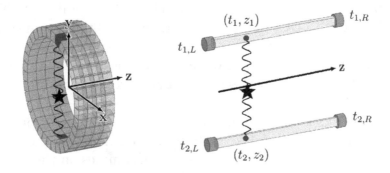

Figure 2.4. Comparison of position reconstruction in state-of-the-art PET scanner based
on inorganic crystals (left part) and the J-PET scanner (right part). The figure is adapted
from [44].

In general, the J-PET tomograph registers the information about each
coincidence of two γ photons in the form of indices of a pair of scintillator strips, and photons time of arrival on each of the photomultipliers
attached to the strips denoted with $t_{1,L}; t_{1,R}; t_{2,L}; t_{2,R}$, where subscripts
L and R indicate the left and the right side of the strip, respectively.
In the case of a classical PET scanner, the information about indices of
pair of crystals is sufficient to indicate correct LOR, i.e., the uncertainty
of estimated position of interaction of each γ photon with the crystal
detector is limited by the size of crystals (see left part in Fig. 2.4). On
the other hand, in the J-PET scanner, position z_1 (z_2) of γ photon interaction along the strip is determined based on time difference measured
on both sides of the scintillator strip $t_{1,L} - t_{1,R}$ ($t_{2,L} - t_{2,R}$). The time
of the interaction (hit-time) of γ photon in the strip t_1 (t_2) is estimated
as an arithmetic mean of times at left $t_{1,L}$ ($t_{2,L}$) and right $t_{1,R}$ ($t_{2,R}$) side
of the plastic scintillator. Therefore, the time resolution of the J-PET
scanner determines not only the uncertainty of position reconstruction
along the LOR, as in case of the conventional PET systems, but also
has an impact on the uncertainty of position reconstruction along the
scintillator strip. For example for plastic strips with the length of 30 cm,

the time resolution of moment of interaction amounts to about 190 ps (FWHM) [17]. This translates to the axial position resolution of about 2.3 cm (FWHM) and resolution in the determination of the annihilation point along LOR of about 3.2 cm (FWHM).

The unique geometry and scintillation materials applied in the J-PET scanner require specialized electronics capable of measuring time with extremely high precision. Current prototype electronics is based on Field-Programmable Gate Array (FPGA) units hosting several dozen Time-to-Digital Converter (TDC) modules [47]. Each TDC module measures the time of arrival and the width of analog signals with a time resolution of 12 ps [48]. Exact description of the electronics system applied in the J-PET detector is beyond the scope of this work; the interested reader is referred to [49, 50].

The analog signals are sampled in the voltage domain at pre-specified number of thresholds by the dedicated FPGA based Multi-Voltage Threshold unit [51]. This results in vector of samples on the leading and trailing edges of the analog signal and opens new perspectives of recovering the original signal waveform. This problem is of main importance in case of the J-PET as the timing information influences the accuracy of time and position reconstruction. The topic of signal recovery and position reconstruction, denoted through this work as low-level processing, will be discussed in detail in chapter 4. Moreover, the extremely high precision of time measurement allows to investigate a completely new approach to image processing. In particular, precise TOF information enables a development of a PET image reconstruction algorithm that operates exclusively in the image space. The novel concepts of high-level image processing described throughout this work will be discussed in detail in chapter 5.

3. Algorithmic background

This chapter presents methods that constitute the theoretical background for digital signal and image processing proposed in this work. The algorithms described on the following pages are essential for formulation and solution of subsequent steps of signal and image processing in the J-PET detector. For clarity of the presentation, state-of-the-art data processing methods are presented separately. Details of the applications and modifications of algorithms described in this part will be introduced in chapters 4 and 5.

The methods described in this chapter are applied to different type of data, depending on the stage of data processing. Despite the fact that the details of the signal and image processing in the J-PET scanner will be explained and discussed in chapters 4 and 5, at this point I would like to underline a few important aspects. First of all, it should be stressed that Compressive Sensing (CS) theory is the key method in the proposed signal recovery scheme. The idea of the CS approach will be introduced in section 3.1. Moreover, one of the most important aspect of the proposed image reconstruction is the application of Total Variation (TV) regularization. The concept of the TV regularization will be discussed in section 3.2. Finally, the visualization of the feature space of the information acquired by the J-PET scanner is provided by using the Self-Organizing Maps (SOMs). The short introduction to unsupervised learning algorithms will be given in section 3.3.

3.1 Compressive Sensing

The CS [52, 53] is a signal processing method that exploits the sparsity of a signal to recover it from far fewer samples than required by the Nyquist–Shannon sampling theorem. Consider the recovery of a finite signal $y^0 \in \mathbb{R}^N$ in a situation where the number M of available samples, denoted as measurement $y_\Omega \in \mathbb{R}^M$, is much smaller than the signal dimension N (y_Ω is sampled on some partial subset Ω, where the cardinality $|\Omega| = M$). In the CS method, a sparse expansion $x^0 \in \mathbb{R}^N$ of signal y^0, evaluated via linear and orthonormal transformation $y^0 = Ax^0$, is considered. In the following we assume that we are given a contaminated measurement y_Ω and hence:

$$y_\Omega = A_\Omega x^0 + e \qquad (3.1)$$

where A_Ω is a $M \times N$ matrix modeling the sampling system, constructed from M rows of matrix A that corresponds to the indexes of y_Ω described in the subset Ω, and e is an error term. It should be stressed that in the case of presence of noise, represented by signal e, instead of an exact recovery of signal x^0 we will consider the solution $\hat{x}$, and by analogy, instead of signal y^0 we will consider the solution $\hat{y}$. The CS method is an attempt to recover $\hat{x}$ by solving optimization problems of the form

$$\hat{x} = \arg\min ||x||_1 \quad \text{such that} \quad ||y_\Omega - A_\Omega x||_2 \le \epsilon \qquad (3.2)$$

where ϵ is the size of the error term e. The l_1 minimization approach provides a powerful framework for recovering sparse signals. Moreover, the use of l_1 minimization leads to convex optimization problems for which there exist a variety of greedy approaches like Orthogonal Matching Pursuit [54] or Basis Pursuit [55]. Other insights provided by CS are related to the construction of measurement matrices (A_Ω) that satisfy the Restricted Isometry Property [56, 57]. For an extensive review of CS the reader is referred to [52, 53, 56, 57].

3.2   Total Variation regularization

The most common class of regularization methods in image processing is based on TV approach [58]. The TV-norm of 3-dimensional image $\mathbf{f}$ can be defined either as the anisotropic norm:

$$\mathrm{TV}_1(\mathbf{f}) = \sum_i \left(|D_i^{(x)}\mathbf{f}| + |D_i^{(y)}\mathbf{f}| + |D_i^{(z)}\mathbf{f}| \right) \qquad (3.3)$$

or the isotropic norm:

$$\mathrm{TV}_2(\mathbf{f}) = \sum_i \sqrt{\left(D_i^{(x)}\mathbf{f}\right)^2 + \left(D_i^{(y)}\mathbf{f}\right)^2 + \left(D_i^{(z)}\mathbf{f}\right)^2} \qquad (3.4)$$

where $D^{(x)} \in \mathbb{R}^{N \times N}$, $D^{(y)} \in \mathbb{R}^{N \times N}$ and $D^{(z)} \in \mathbb{R}^{N \times N}$ are the first-order forward finite-difference operators, that approximate the gradient operators along the x, y, z directions, respectively. Therefore, $D_i^{(u)}\mathbf{f} \in \mathbb{R}$ is the discrete gradient of the image at pixel i along the u direction ($u = x, y, z$). In this work only the isotropic case, $\mathrm{TV} \triangleq \mathrm{TV}_2$, will be considered, however the treatment for the anisotropic case is completely analogous. We define $D = \left(D^{(x)}; D^{(y)}; D^{(z)} \right) \in \mathbb{R}^{3N \times N}$ as the total first-order forward finite-difference operator. Thus, the TV norm in Eq. (3.4) can be expressed as:

$$\text{TV}(\mathbf{f}) = \sum_i \|D_i \mathbf{f}\|_2 \qquad (3.5)$$

where $D_i \mathbf{f} \in \mathbb{R}^3$ is the discrete gradient of the image at pixel i.

Consider a linear system of equations

$$\mathbf{b} = A\mathbf{f}. \qquad (3.6)$$

If the measurement $\mathbf{b}$ is contaminated with noise, optimization algorithms find a solution $\mathbf{f}$ of Eq. (3.6) by solving an unconstrained problem:

$$\min_{\mathbf{f}} \ \text{TV}(\mathbf{f}) + \frac{\mu}{2}\|A\mathbf{f} - \mathbf{b}\|_2^2, \qquad (3.7)$$

or a closely related constrained problem:

$$\min_{\mathbf{f}} \ \text{TV}(\mathbf{f}) \quad \text{subject to} \quad \|A\mathbf{f} - \mathbf{b}\|_2 \leq \epsilon, \qquad (3.8)$$

where μ and ϵ are the regularization parameters. The computational challenges arise from the fact that applications are invariably large-scale. For example, the measurement matrix A for an $256 \times 256 \times 256$ image, stored as a vector $\mathbf{f}$ with 16777216 entries, is 16777216×16777216, making the system far too large to solve or even store explicitly. For a class of spatially invariant image reconstruction problems, the matrix A is a block-circulant matrix [59]. Therefore, Fourier transforms can be utilized to efficiently find a solution. As a result, a huge gain in speed can be realized. In the following we will briefly introduce the unconstrained optimization approach for block-circulant matrix A.

3.2.1 Unconstrained TV regularization problem

The TV minimization problem defined in Eq. (3.7) with definition of TV norm given in Eq. (3.5) may be expressed as:

$$\min_{\mathbf{f}} \ \sum_{i=1}^{N} \|D_i \mathbf{f}\|_2 + \frac{\mu}{2}\|A\mathbf{f} - \mathbf{b}\|_2^2. \qquad (3.9)$$

The problem in Eq. (3.9) is convex, but due to the nondifferentiability and nonlinearity of the TV function, the model is computationally difficult to solve. The first step of solving the problem in Eq. (3.9) is the introduction of an auxiliary variable $\mathbf{w}_i \in \mathbb{R}^3$ to transfer $D_i\mathbf{f}$ out of the nondifferentiable term $\|\cdot\|_2$

$$\min_{\mathbf{f},\mathbf{w}} \sum_{i=1}^{N} \|\mathbf{w}_i\|_2 + \frac{\mu}{2}\|A\mathbf{f} - \mathbf{b}\|_2^2 \quad \text{subject to} \quad D_i\mathbf{f} = \mathbf{w}_i \qquad (3.10)$$

The Lagrangian function $\mathcal{L}(\mathbf{f},\mathbf{w},\lambda)$ of problem in Eq. (3.10) is defined as:

$$\mathcal{L}(\mathbf{f},\mathbf{w},\lambda) = \sum_{i}\left(\|\mathbf{w}_i\|_2 + \lambda_i\left(D_i\mathbf{f} - \mathbf{w}_i\right)\right) + \frac{\mu}{2}\|A\mathbf{f} - \mathbf{b}\|_2^2 \qquad (3.11)$$

where λ_i is the Lagrange multiplier associated with the constraint $D_i\mathbf{f} = \mathbf{w}_i$. According to the idea of the quadratic penalty method, it is likely to penalize the violation of constraint $D_i\mathbf{f} = \mathbf{w}_i$. For instance, one may solve the following problem:

$$\mathcal{L}_A(\mathbf{f},\mathbf{w},\lambda) = \mathcal{L}(\mathbf{f},\mathbf{w},\lambda) + \sum_{i}\left(\frac{\beta}{2}\|D_i\mathbf{f} - \mathbf{w}_i\|_2^2\right) \qquad (3.12)$$

where β is a regularization parameter associated with each quadratic penalty term $\|D_i\mathbf{f} - \mathbf{w}_i\|_2^2$. Minimizing the problem in Eq. (3.12) is known as an augmented Lagrangian method [60, 61]. When the original problem, defined in Eq. (3.9), is convex, the first-order optimality conditions of augmented Lagrangian function become sufficient for finding optimal solution $\mathbf{f}$.

The advantage of the introduction of an auxiliary variable $\mathbf{w}$ is that, while either one of the variables $(\mathbf{f},\mathbf{w})$ is fixed, minimizing the function $\mathcal{L}_A$ with respect to the other has a closed-form formula with low computational complexity. To this end, the alternating direction method is used to iteratively solve the optimization problem in Eq. (3.12).

For a fixed $\mathbf{f}$, all the terms associated with $\mathcal{L}(\mathbf{f},\mathbf{w},\lambda)$ in Eq. (3.12) are separable with respect to $\mathbf{w}_i$, so minimizing for $\mathbf{w}$ is equivalent to solving for $i = 1, \ldots, N$,

$$\min_{\mathbf{w}_i} \|\mathbf{w}_i\|_2 + \lambda_i\left(D_i\mathbf{f} - \mathbf{w}_i\right) + \frac{\beta}{2}\|D_i\mathbf{f} - \mathbf{w}_i\|_2^2, \qquad (3.13)$$

for which the unique minimizer can be found using a shrinkage formula [62]:

$$\mathbf{w}_i = \max\left(\|D_i\mathbf{f} + \frac{\lambda_i}{\beta}\|_2 - \frac{1}{\beta}, 0\right)\frac{D_i\mathbf{f} + \frac{\lambda_i}{\beta}}{\|D_i\mathbf{f} + \frac{\lambda_i}{\beta}\|_2}, \qquad (3.14)$$

where all operations are done component-wise.

On the other hand, for a fixed $\mathbf{w}$, the problem in Eq. (3.12) is quadratic in $\mathbf{f}$ and the solution is given by the normal equation:

$$\left(\mu A^T A + \beta D^T D\right) \mathbf{f} = \mu A^T \mathbf{b} + \beta D^T \mathbf{w} + D^T \lambda. \qquad (3.15)$$

Under the periodic boundary condition for $\mathbf{f}$, $D^T D$, and assuming that the matrix A is a block-circulant, the Hessian matrix

$$H = \mu A^T A + \beta D^T D$$

on the left-hand side of the Eq. (3.15) is circulant and can be diagonalized by discrete Fourier transform (DFT) matrices [59]. Therefore, Eq. (3.15) has the following solution:

$$\mathbf{f} = F \Lambda^{-1} F^{-1} \left(\mu A^T \mathbf{b} + \beta D^T \mathbf{w} + D^T \lambda\right), \qquad (3.16)$$

where F denotes the DFT matrix and Λ is a diagonal matrix storing the eigenvalues of H, i.e., $\Lambda = F^{-1} H F$. It should be underlined that the matrix Λ can be calculated only once, outside of the main loop.

3.3   Self-Organized Maps

The SOM is a technique that provides a way to visualize the high-dimensional data on a two-dimensional map that preserves the most important relations and helps to see the similarity between the clusters of data samples. The SOM is a vector quantization method which places the prototype vectors on a regular low-dimensional grid [63]. The principal goal of a SOM is to transform input data into a 2-dimensional discrete map. An example of SOM is shown in Fig. 3.1. The 2-dimensional synthetic, banana-shaped data set is marked with gray crosses and positions of neurons are marked with black circles. In example in Fig. 3.1a, the network is initialized linearly along the greatest eigenvectors of the training data. Each SOM neuron is associated with a weight vector, which is a position in the input space. Moreover, each neuron has its own map address, which is a fixed position on the grid. Training of the map relies on moving weight vectors (black circles) toward the input data (gray crosses) without spoiling the topology. The map of weight vectors (black circles) is searched to find the neuron whose weight vector is most similar to the input data (x). This neuron is called the best matching unit (BMU). The appropriate weight update equation for neuron i is

$$\Delta w_i = \eta \cdot T(i,j) \cdot (x - w_i) \qquad (3.17)$$

where η is a monotonically decreasing learning coefficient, j is the index of the BMU for the input data x, and $T(i, j)$ is the neighborhood function which gives the distance between the neuron i and the BMU. In the simplest form, the neighbourhood function equals 1 for all neurons close enough to BMU and 0 for others. The most common possibilities are to apply a Gaussian, or mexican-hat functions. However, regardless of the functional form, the neighborhood function shrinks with time.

The learning process is repeated for each input data in data set for a large number of epochs. Trained SOM network describes a mapping from an input space to a 2-dimensional map space (see Fig. 3.1b in this example). Once trained, the map can classify a vector from the input space by finding the neuron with the closest weight vector to the input space vector.

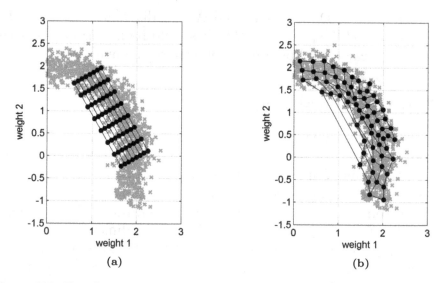

(a)   (b)

Figure 3.1. Visualization of banana-shaped data set by 2-dimensional SOM. The arrangement of neurons (black circles) correspond to a situation before (a) and after (b) training of the network.

4. Low-level data processing in Jagiellonian PET

This chapter describes the subsequent steps of low-level data processing in the J-PET scanner. The goal of low-level reconstruction is an evaluation of time and position of each particular event of positron emission. A simple setup with two detection modules that permits the reconstruction of information about an event is shown in Fig. 4.1.

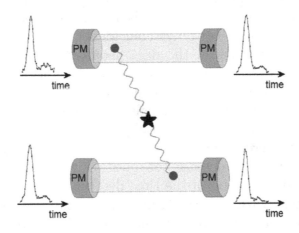

Figure 4.1. Schematic view of the data registration in J-PET detector. The reconstruction of positron emission event, marked with black star, requires the information about four electric signals arrival to the left and right photomultipliers (PMs) of the two modules that register in coincidence.

A single detection module consists of a long scintillator strip and a pair of photomultipliers (PMs) attached to opposite ends of the strip (see Fig. 4.1). The subsequent steps of the reconstruction take place in the reverse order than the physical processes of interactions in the detector. Light pulses produced in the strip propagate to its edges where they are converted via photomultipliers into electric signals. Measurement of electric signals results in timestamps from both sides of each scintillator, allowing the extraction of timing, position and energy information for each γ photon interaction marked with gray circle in Fig. 4.1. The time and position of the γ photon interaction in the scintillator strip is calculated based on times at left ($t_{(L)}$) and right ($t_{(R)}$) side of the strip. In the first approximation, the time of interaction may be estimated as an arithmetic mean of $t_{(L)}$ and $t_{(R)}$ and the position of interaction along the strip may be calculated as ($t_{(L)} - t_{(R)})v_{sc}/2$, where v_{sc} denotes the speed of light signals in the scintillator strip. The energy deposited in the scintillator strip may be expressed in terms of the number of photoelectrons registered by the photomultipliers and is proportional to the arithmetic mean of a number of photoelectrons registered at the left and right sides of the scintillator; the value of energy calibration factor was evaluated in [17]. The registration of single event of positron emission, used for the image reconstruction, is based on the detection of both γ photons in two modules in a narrow time window. Therefore, a single image-building event, marked with black star in Fig. 4.1, includes information about four times of light signals arrival to the left and right ends of the two modules that register in coincidence.

The two main features of the data acquired in the J-PET scanner that have the greatest impact on the TOF resolution are: (i) a very short rise-time and duration of the signals and (ii) a relation between the shape and amplitude of the signals and the hit position. The latter feature usually distorts the time resolution but, when the waveform of the signal is registered, the information about a change of the shape with the position may increase the position resolution and indirectly improve also the resolution of the time determination [64]. However, to probe the signals, with duration times of few nanoseconds, a sampling time in the order of picoseconds is required. This can be done well with the oscilloscopes during laboratory studies on the prototype, but in the final multimodular devices with hundreds of photomultipliers, probing with oscilloscopes is not feasible [65]. On the other hand, an application of the typical techniques for time measurement, based on a single-level leading-edge discriminators, is not sufficient and prevents achieving the best timing properties of the J-PET detector. In chapter 2, a multi-threshold sampling method to generate samples of a PET event waveform was proposed as a solution to this problem and then implemented in the J-PET scanner [51].

This chapter is organized as follows. In section 4.1, we will start with the introduction of the model of signal waveform registered on photomultiplier output. Next, we will define the problem of signal recovery and derive briefly the modified Tikhonov regularization method in section 4.2. In the last part of this section we will introduce the theorem enabling the determination of the signal recovery error as a function of the number of samples. In section 4.3, we will describe the method for reconstruction of γ photon interaction position in the scintillator strip. The method can be applied to both raw samples registered in the voltage domain and recovered waveforms of the signal, therefore allowing the comparison of the spatial resolutions evaluated based on different representation of data. The last study presented in this chapter, in section 4.4, will concern the prediction of theoretical time resolution of the J-PET detector.

4.1 Model of signal waveform registered on photomultiplier

We assume that the γ photon interacts in the scintillator strip at time Θ^0 and in the position z^0. The time of the photon registration at the photomultiplier, referred to as t_r, is considered as a random variable, equal to the sum of three contributing values:

$$t_r = t_e + t_p + t_d, \tag{4.1}$$

where t_e is the photon emission time, t_p is the propagation time of the photon along the scintillator strip and t_d is the photomultiplier transit time. Assuming that the times t_e, t_p, t_d, given in Eq. (4.1), are independent random variables with probability density functions (pdfs) denoted with $f_{t_e}, f_{t_p}, f_{t_d}$, respectively, the distribution function of t_r is given as the convolution:

$$f_{t_r}(t) = (f_{t_e} * f_{t_p} * f_{t_d})(t), \quad t > 0.$$

In case of the ternary plastic scintillators used in the J-PET detector [32], the distribution of t_e is well approximated by the following formula [66, 67]:

$$f_{t_e}(t) = \kappa_e \int_{\Theta^0}^{t} \left(e^{-\frac{t-\tau}{\tau_d}} - e^{-\frac{t-\tau}{\tau_r}} \right) e^{-\frac{(\tau - \Theta^0 - 2.5\sigma_e)^2}{2\sigma_e^2}} d\tau, \tag{4.2}$$

where $\tau_d = 1.5$ ns, $\tau_r = 0.005$ ns and $\sigma_e = 0.2$ ns, and κ_e stands for the normalization constant. The values of the parameters τ_d, τ_r, σ_e were adjusted in order to describe the properties of the light pulses from the BC-420 scintillator [19]. By definition in Eq. (4.2):

$$t_e \geq \Theta^0. \tag{4.3}$$

Initial direction of flight of the photon in the scintillator is uniformly distributed. The photon on its way along the scintillator strip from the emission point to the photomultiplier may undergo many internal reflections whose number depends on the scintillator's geometry and the photon's emission angle. However, the space reflection symmetries of the cuboidal shapes, considered in this thesis, enables a significant simplification of the photon transport algorithm, without following photon propagation in a typical manner. The statistical modelling of this phenomena was presented in details in Ref. [19] and the analytical function describing the distribution function f_{t_p} may be expressed by the following formula:

$$f_{t_p}(t) = \frac{\kappa_p \cdot z^0}{t^2} \cdot e^{-\mu_{\text{eff}} \cdot v_{\text{sc}} \cdot t}, \tag{4.4}$$

where v_{sc} is the speed of light in the scintillator strip, μ_{eff} is the effective absorption coefficient for the scintillator material and κ_p the normalization constant. The $0 \leq z^0 \leq L_d$ is the longitudinal position of the emission point, where L_d is the detector length. The pdf function $f_{t_p}(t)$ in Eq. (4.4) is nonzero only for:

$$t_p \geq \frac{z^0}{v_{\text{sc}}}, \tag{4.5}$$

where $t_p = \frac{z^0}{v_{\text{sc}}}$ corresponds to the photon flying along the strip. Finally, the time of registration t_r is smeared using Gaussian distribution centered on the mean transition time T_d and variance σ_d^2 estimated empirically:

$$f_{t_d}(t) = \frac{1}{\sqrt{2\pi}\sigma_d} \exp\left(-\frac{(t - T_d)^2}{\sigma_d^2}\right). \tag{4.6}$$

In this work, we assume that the signal registered at the photomultiplier output has the same functional dependence on the time as the f_{t_r} function. We assume that the signal $y \in \mathbb{R}^N$ is discretized by the oscilloscope. It is sampled in the constant time intervals denoted with T_s. From the conditions Eq. (4.3) and (4.5), it follows that the registration time t_r fulfils the inequality:

$$t_r \geq \Theta^0 + \frac{z^0}{v_{\text{sc}}}.$$

It was assumed that the transition time $t_d \geq 0$. Therefore, the nth time sample is given by:

$$t^{(n)} = nT_s + \Theta^0 + \frac{z^0}{v_{\text{sc}}} \qquad n = 1, 2, ..., N, \tag{4.7}$$

and the nth sample of the signal y is given as:

$$y(n) = \beta(E, z^0) \cdot f_n, \quad \text{where} \quad f_n = f_{t_r}(t^{(n)}) \qquad n = 1, 2, ..., N, \quad (4.8)$$

where $\beta(E, z^0)$ is a coefficient providing the scaling of the pdf function f_{t_r} in order to obtain the voltage signal:

$$\beta(E, z^0) = \beta_E \cdot \beta_z.$$

The value of $\beta(E, z^0)$ depends on the energy deposited in the plastic scintillator during the γ photon interaction (β_E factor) and on the position of the γ photon interaction along the strip (β_z factor). The higher the value of deposited energy, the higher the value of β_E parameter and higher the signal amplitude. The β_z is necessary to describe absorption of photons propagating through the scintillator strip, since f_{t_p} provides only information about the shape of the signal (see Eq. (4.4)). Contributions of β_E to β are the same for both ends of the strip but β_z are different. Hereon, in order to simplify the notation of the parameter $\beta(E, z^0)$, we use only the symbol β.

We add a random noise term $v_{(L,R)}$ to the signal $y_{(L,R)}$ at the left (L) and right (R) end of the strip. Hence registered signals $\hat{y}_{(L)}$ and $\hat{y}_{(R)}$ may be expressed as[1]:

$$\hat{y}_{(L)}(\Theta^0, z^0) = y_{(L)}(\Theta^0, z^0) + v_{(L)}. \qquad (4.9)$$

$$\hat{y}_{(R)}(\Theta^0, z^0) = y_{(R)}(\Theta^0, z^0) + v_{(R)}. \qquad (4.10)$$

We assume that the noise $v_{(L)}$ and $v_{(R)}$ are uncorrelated and obey the same multivariate normal distribution:

$$v_{(L)}, v_{(R)} \sim \mathcal{N}(0, S), \qquad (4.11)$$

where S is the covariance matrix of $\hat{y}_{(L)}$ and $\hat{y}_{(R)}$. The noise contribution to the signals registered on the left ($\hat{y}_{(L)}$) and right ($\hat{y}_{(R)}$) side of the scintillator strip is the same, and therefore we will skip the L, R indices in further analysis. We assume that the noise signal v is defined as a sum of two components:

$$v = v_p + v_r, \qquad (4.12)$$

where v_p describes the perturbations of the pdf function f_{t_r}, based on limited number of input photon signals, and v_r stands for the signal recovery noise. The latter component is introduced by the procedure

---

[1] L. Raczyński et al., Calculation of the time resolution of the J-PET tomograph using kernel density estimation, *Phys. Med. Biol.* **62** (2017) 5078−5080.

of signal recovery based on the limited number of registered samples of the signal in the voltage domain. The problem of signal recovery was introduced in Ref. [2] and will be discussed in section 4.2. We assume that the noises v_p and v_r are uncorrelated and normally distributed with covariance matrices S_p and S_r, respectively. Thus, one may write that:

$$S = S_p + S_r. \tag{4.13}$$

The exact values of v_p and v_r depend on the type of the photomultiplier applied. The J-PET tomograph can be equipped with various types of photomultiplier:

- PMT – vacuum tube photomultiplier (standard in the J-PET prototype),

- SiPM – silicon photomultiplier,

- MCP – microchannel plates photomultiplier.

In case of vacuum tube or silicon photomultipliers, registration of the whole signal is not feasible, and therefore sampling in the voltage domain using a predefined number of voltage levels is needed. The microchannel plate photomultipliers are the most promising for application in the J-PET instrument due to the possibility of direct registration of the timestamp of each single photon. It is worth noting that v_r vanishes in the case of MCP photomultiplier; there is no need to recover the output signal since all arrival times of photons are registered.[2]

4.2 Recovery of signal waveform based on limited number of samples

It is evident that the time and spatial resolutions of the J-PET scanner depend on the number of threshold levels of an electronic system for probing the signals in a voltage domain. However, the number of channels in the electronic devices is a very important factor in determining the cost of the PET scanner. Therefore, the question arises: is it possible to recover the whole signal based on only a few samples? Equivalently, how many threshold levels have to be applied to achieve a reasonable estimation error?

In this section we propose a novel signal recovery scheme based on ideas from the Tikhonov regularization [68, 69] and CS methods that is

---

[2] L. Raczyński et al., Calculation of the time resolution of the J-PET tomograph using kernel density estimation, *Phys. Med. Biol.* **62** (2017) 5082–5083.

compatible with the signal processing scenario in J-PET devices. The most important part of our investigations is to determine a dependence of the signal recovery error on the number of samples taken in the voltage domain. In this section the formula for calculations of the recovery error will be introduced and proven.

As in the CS framework, we wish to recover a finite signal $\hat{y} \in \mathbb{R}^N$ given a contaminated measurement $y_\Omega \in \mathbb{R}^M$ sampled on some partial subset Ω, where the cardinality $|\Omega| = M$ (for details see section 3.1). The evaluation of $\hat{y}$ requires two steps: i) recovery of the sparse expansion $\hat{x}$ and ii) calculation of $\hat{y}$ based on the $\hat{x}$. The first step of the procedure is crucial. In the case discussed in this work, the matrix A transforming the sparse expansion $\hat{x}$ into the signal $\hat{y}$ is evaluated based on the Principal Component Analysis (PCA) decomposition [70] of the training set of fully sampled signals. Under the assumption that signals in both spaces are given with multivariate normal distributions (MVN), the solution $\hat{x}$ may be found as the minimizer of the following expression:

$$\hat{x} = \arg\min\{(y_\Omega - A_\Omega x)^T R^{-1}(y_\Omega - A_\Omega x) + (x - m_x)^T P^{-1}(x - m_x)\}. \quad (4.14)$$

The formula proposed in Eq. (4.14) describes a modified Tikhonov regularization (TR) method [68,69], where additionally an information about prior distribution of the solution x is applied in second term. The parameters m_x and P are the mean value and covariance matrix of a dataset X that describes the prior distribution, respectively. The dataset X is evaluated based on the PCA decomposition of training signals stored in matrix Y, i.e.,

$$X = A^T Y. \quad (4.15)$$

The matrix A in Eq. (4.15) is calculated in such a way that the projection of the data matrix Y with successive basis vectors inherits the greatest possible variance in the data set Y. Thus, the values on diagonal in the covariance matrix P are sorted in non-increasing order. The parameters $A_\Omega x$ and R in Eq. (4.14) are the mean value and covariance matrix of a measured signal y_Ω, respectively. The covariance matrix R is diagonal with the values on the diagonal equal to the measurement error variances σ^2.

Beside the advantage of including the additional information from training signals, a further benefit of the TR approach is that the problem in Eq. (4.14) has an optimal solution which can be determined explicitly. The derivation of the solution of a sparse solution $\hat{x}$, and its covariance matrix, denoted as S_r (see Eq. (4.13)), for a particular measurement y_Ω, is based on Refs. [68, 69, 71]:

$$\hat{x} = (P^{-1}m_x + A_\Omega^T R^{-1} y_\Omega) \cdot (P^{-1} + A_\Omega^T R^{-1} A_\Omega)^{-1}, \qquad (4.16)$$

$$S_r = (P^{-1} + A_\Omega^T R^{-1} A_\Omega)^{-1}. \qquad (4.17)$$

It is worth noting that the solutions in Eq. (4.16) and (4.17) are analogous to Kalman filter update equations (cf. Refs. [72, 73]). It should be stressed that the parameters of PCA decomposition are calculated only once, at the preparation stage of the procedure. Thus, the same matrices A, P and vector m_x, are used to recover a signal $\hat{x}$ for each measurement in Eq. (4.16). However, the evaluation of the covariance matrix S_r, according to Eq. (4.17), does not require the information about the measurement y_Ω, and may be provided at the preparation stage. This fact opens a possibility for an estimation of the theoretical value of the recovery error. This idea will be presented in the next section.

4.2.1   Calculation of recovery error

One of the benefits of using the TR approach is that it provides an easy way to obtain the error term of the recovered signal $\hat{y}$. Since the matrix A is orthonormal, we have

$$||\hat{y} - y^0||_2^2 = ||\hat{x} - x^0||_2^2, \qquad (4.18)$$

and therefore we may focus on the recovered signal $\hat{x}$ error. In multivariate statistics, the trace of the covariance matrix is considered as the total variance. We will denote the trace of covariance matrix S_r as σ_x^2. It is worth noting that σ_x^2 is the mean value of the recovery error squared norm $||\hat{x} - x^0||_2^2$. Let $P(k)$ be the kth diagonal element of covariance matrix P. We find the smallest value of D, and the largest value of τ (with constraints $D > 0$ and $\tau > 0$) such that for each $1 \leq k \leq N$:

$$P(k) \leq D \cdot e^{-\tau k}. \qquad (4.19)$$

From Eq. (4.19) one may see that τ controls the decrease rate of $P(k)$: the greater τ, the faster the decreasing of $P(k)$ and better the compressibility of signal x. The characteristics D and τ of the prior distribution of signal x and a standard deviation of noise (σ) enable us to provide the formula for average value of the recovery error σ_x^2. For this purpose we formulate the following theorem:

Theorem. *Suppose that D and τ describe the decrease rate of variances of signal x according to Eq. (4.19). The signal x may be recovered as the solution to Eq. (4.16) with an average value of error*

$$\sigma_x^2 \approx \frac{\sigma^2 N}{M\tau} \log\left(\frac{\sigma^2 N + MD}{\sigma^2 N}\right). \qquad (4.20)$$

Equation (4.20) enables us to estimate the number of required samples M of signal to achieve a preselected mean recovery error. Intuitively, the σ_x^2 is also closely related to the compressibility of signal x, and from Eq. (4.20) one may observe that an average recovery error is inversely proportional to the constant value τ. The proof of the theorem is given in the appendix A.1.

4.3 Reconstruction of γ photon interaction position in scintillator

In this section we describe a concept of reconstruction of the γ photon hit position. The method is based on the statistical model of signals [1]. The algorithm may be applied to different representations of the data: to raw signal probed in the voltage domain and fully recovered signals based on the idea introduced in section 4.2. The description given in this section includes an explanation of the methods used for the test of the normality of data and determination of the effective number of degrees of freedom.

The method of hit-position reconstruction consists of two steps. First, the scintillator's volume is discretized and for each bin a high statistics set of reference signals is created. The objective of the second part of the procedure is to qualify the new measurement to one of the given sets of signals and hence determine the hit position. The shapes of the signals depend on the hit position and can be used for its reconstruction.

Consider L data sets $G^{(i)}$, where $i = 1, ..., L$. Each $G^{(i)}$ is a $M_i \times N_i$ matrix of vectors representing signals gathered for the ith position; M_i is the number of the collected signals and N_i stands for vector's dimension equal to the number of samples per signal. In practice, all signals have the same dimension and $N_i = N$ for all i. The jth signal in the ith data set corresponds to the jth row of the matrix $G^{(i)}$ and is denoted by the vector $G_j^{(i)}$. If the measured coordinates of vectors in all L data sets are normally distributed then the mean value m_i and covariance matrix C_i of the data set $G^{(i)}$ describe it completely. Assuming their normality, the proposed reconstruction procedure qualifies a new measurement, represented by vector u, to one of the data sets $G^{(i)}$ by using the Mahalanobis distances $d^{(i)}$ between u and m_i:

$$d^{(i)} = (u - m_i)C_i^{-1}(u - m_i)^{\mathrm{T}} \qquad i = 1, 2, ..., L. \qquad (4.21)$$

The measured signal u is qualified to the data set $\hat{i}$ with the smallest distance $d^{(i)}$:

$$\hat{i} = \arg\min d^{(i)}. \qquad (4.22)$$

4.3.1   Test of normality of the data

There are numerous procedures for testing whether multivariate vectors from a given dataset have a MVN distribution [74–77]. We propose an alternative procedure for testing a MVN distribution as an extension of statistical test based on q-q approach [78]. In order to verify normality of the dataset in $G^{(i)}$, the observations squared Mahalanobis distances for M_i vectors from $G^{(i)}$ data set are calculated:

$$d_j^{(i)} = (G_j^{(i)} - m_i)C_i^{-1}(G_j^{(i)} - m_i)^{\mathrm{T}} \qquad j = 1, 2, ..., M_i. \qquad (4.23)$$

where m_i, and C_i are estimated based on the data set S_i. In [79] authors assumed that the evaluated distances in Eq. (4.23) have a χ^2 distribution with N degrees of freedom. In the following we will show that this is not necessarily the case, and the number of effective degrees of freedom may be smaller due to signal correlation. The discussion about the effective number of degrees of freedom, denoted hereafter as V, will be given in section 4.3.2.

We provide a statistical test for data set $G^{(i)}$ by comparing the distribution of $d_j^{(i)}$ defined in Eq. (4.23) with the theoretical χ^2 distribution with V degrees of freedom. The normalization of theoretical histogram is provided to ensure that sum of counts in both histograms is the same and equal to M_i. We apply uneven bin size, in order to store in each bin of the theoretical χ^2 histogram a constant number of counts F_T. In the calculations, we have selected $F_T = 30$, and therefore the Poisson distribution may be approximated accurately by the normal distribution. Hence, we compare the two histograms via statistical test r defined as follows:

$$r_i(V) = \sum_{k=1}^{B_i} \frac{(F_k^{(i)} - F_T)^2}{F_T}, \qquad (4.24)$$

where $F_k^{(i)}$ value is the number of counts in the kth bin in the experimental histogram from the ith data set, and $B_i = M_i/F_T$ is the number of bins in the histograms. The bin sizes were calculated from the theoretical χ^2 with V degrees of freedom. The test statistic r_i is a χ^2 random variable with mean B_i and standard deviation $\sqrt{2B_i}$; owing to well known concentration inequalities, the probability that r_i exceeds its mean plus three standard deviations is small. In the following we will find the parameter λ that fulfills the equation:

$$r_i(V) = B_i + \lambda\sqrt{2B_i}, \tag{4.25}$$

and we state that the null hypothesis that the experimental histogram has a χ^2 distribution with V degrees of freedom is true, if $\lambda < 3$.

4.3.2 Number of effective degrees of freedom

Components of the signal vector are mutually correlated in a complicated manner so the effective V has to be determined empirically. Its upper bound $V_{\max}$ is equal to the number of independent variables N. In order to determine the minimal $V_{\min}$, the diagonalization of the covariance matrix C_i of each data set $G^{(i)}$ is performed. The diagonalized covariance matrix, denoted with $\hat{C}_i$, has values on diagonal sorted in non-increasing order. We define the parameter ρ as a normalized sum of k variances on the diagonal of $\hat{C}_i$,

$$\rho_k = \mathbb{1}_k\hat{C}_i\mathbb{1}_k^T(\mathbb{1}_N\hat{C}_i\mathbb{1}_N^T)^{-1}, \tag{4.26}$$

where $\mathbb{1}_k$ is the N-dimensional row vector with ones at positions from 1 to k, and zeros from $k+1$ to N. According to this definition, $\mathbb{1}_N$ is a vector with all N values equal to one. The ρ is a non-decreasing function and we assume that at least $\rho > 0.95$ is necessary to describe data set $G^{(i)}$ properly. The minimal number of variables $V_{\min}$ is equal to the smallest k for which $\rho_k > 0.95$. After the determination of $V_{\min}$, calculations of statistics r are repeated for different V in the range from $V_{\min}$ to $V_{\max}$. The theoretical χ^2 distribution with V degrees of freedom for which the smallest statistics r (see Eq. (4.24)) and hence smaller parameter λ (from Eq. (4.25)) was calculated, is selected. The experimental distribution is said to be a MVN distribution with V degrees of freedom, if λ is smaller than 3.

4.4 Prediction of theoretical resolutions of the J-PET scanner

The last part of the chapter describing the low-level data processing concerns the prediction of theoretical resolutions of the J-PET detector.

Further improvement in the time resolution of the tomograph requires developments in techniques of signal processing and effective parametrizations of detector features. The estimate of the time resolution, presented in this section, is based on statistical properties of the signals in plastic scintillators described in section 4.1. In this section we will introduce the formula for calculations of the time resolution based on the covariance matrix S of the noise signals registered on photomultipliers (see Eq. (4.11) for details).

The reconstructed values of time and position of γ photon interaction are denoted with $\hat{\Theta}$ and $\hat{z}$, respectively. According to the definitions of the theoretical (y) and registered $(\hat{y})$ signals given in section 4.1, the reconstruction of $\hat{\Theta}, \hat{z}$ may be pursued by minimization of the function:

$$W(\Delta\Theta, \Delta z) = (y_{(L)} - \hat{y}_{(L)})(y_{(L)} - \hat{y}_{(L)})^T + (y_{(R)} - \hat{y}_{(R)})(y_{(R)} - \hat{y}_{(R)})^T, \tag{4.27}$$

where:

$$\Delta\Theta = \Theta^0 - \Theta,$$
$$\Delta z = z^0 - z.$$

The solutions $\hat{\Theta}, \hat{z}$ are found as:

$$(\Delta\hat{\Theta}, \Delta\hat{z}) = \arg\min W(\Delta\Theta, \Delta z) \tag{4.28}$$

where hat denotes the estimators. From Eq. (4.27) it is seen that the error function W is a positive-valued random variable. We assume that $\Delta\hat{\Theta}$ has normal distribution:

$$\Delta\hat{\Theta} \sim \mathcal{N}(0, \sigma_\Theta^2), \tag{4.29}$$

with 0 mean value and standard deviation denoted with σ_Θ. Derivation of the time resolution (CRT) based on the σ_Θ will be introduced in section 4.4.2.

In order to calculate the σ_Θ, function W has to be analyzed near the minimum, $(0,0)$. According to Eq. (4.27), the random variable $W(0,0)$ may be expressed as:

$$W(0,0) = v_{(L)} v_{(L)}^T + v_{(R)} v_{(R)}^T,$$
$$= \sum_{n=1}^{N} v_{(L)}^2(n) + v_{(R)}^2(n). \tag{4.30}$$

The variance of W in the minimum will be denoted hereafter as $\text{Var}[W_{\min}]$. Using Eq. (4.11) and assuming the diagonality of matrix S, yields:

$$\text{Var}[W_{\min}] = 2 \sum_{n=1}^{N} 2S^2(n, n). \qquad (4.31)$$

On the other hand, we may analyse the shape of the function W in the two-dimensional space of time $(\Delta\hat{\Theta})$ and position $(\Delta\hat{z})$ errors. In the following, we will consider only the $(\Delta\hat{\Theta})$ error, and therefore analyse W in one dimension $(\Delta\hat{z} = 0)$. Taylor series expansion of W around $(0, 0)$ is given as:

$$W(\Delta\hat{\Theta}, 0) \approx W(0, 0) + \frac{\partial W(0, 0)}{\partial \Delta\hat{\Theta}} \Delta\hat{\Theta} + \frac{1}{2} \cdot \frac{\partial^2 W(0, 0)}{\partial \Delta\hat{\Theta}^2} \Delta\hat{\Theta}^2$$

$$\approx \alpha_0 + \alpha_1 \Delta\hat{\Theta} + \alpha_2 \Delta\hat{\Theta}^2. \qquad (4.32)$$

It is evident that the first two coefficients (α_0, α_1) are equal to zero and the quadratic approximation simplifies to:

$$W(\Delta\hat{\Theta}, 0) \approx \alpha_2 \Delta\hat{\Theta}^2. \qquad (4.33)$$

Under the assumption of normality of $\Delta\hat{\Theta}$ distribution the random variable $W(\Delta\hat{\Theta}, 0)$ given in Eq. (4.33), has a χ^2 distribution with the variance:

$$\text{Var}[W_{\min}] \approx 2\alpha_2{}^2 \sigma_\Theta{}^4. \qquad (4.34)$$

The comparison of two formulas describing the $\text{Var}[W_{\min}]$, in Eq. (4.34) and (4.31), enables us to determine the standard deviation[3]:

$$\sigma_\Theta = \sqrt[4]{\frac{2 \sum_{n=1}^{N} S^2(n, n)}{\alpha_2{}^2}}. \qquad (4.35)$$

The σ_Θ requires evaluation of covariance matrix S and in particular the matrix S_p. Derivation of the matrix S_p will be given in section 4.4.1. Moreover, the estimation of the CRT based on the standard deviation σ_Θ will be provided in section 4.4.2.

4.4.1 Influence of limited number of photons on registered signal error

According to the assumption proposed in section 4.1, the noise in the measured signal contains two components: statistical fluctuations of the

---

[3] L. Raczyński et al., Calculation of the time resolution of the J-PET tomograph using kernel density estimation, *Phys. Med. Biol.* **62** (2017) 5081−5082.

number of photoelectrons registered by the photosensor described with covariance matrix S_p, and the effect of the limited number of samples of the signal in the voltage domain, described with covariance matrix S_r. In section 4.2, a formula for calculating the matrix S_r was introduced and in the following we will determine the matrix S_p.

The registered signal y affected only by the v_p noise will be denoted with:

$$\tilde{y} = y + v_p.$$

The output signal $\tilde{y}$ may be evaluated by using a model of the single photon:

$$\tilde{y} = \sum_{k=1}^{N_p} \tilde{y}_k, \qquad (4.36)$$

where N_p is the number of individual photoelectrons. For all types of photomultipliers we use the Gaussian model [80] for shape of signal of single photoelectron, with the width σ_p :

$$\tilde{y}_k(n) = \frac{\beta}{\sqrt{(2\pi)N_p\sigma_p}} \exp\left(-\frac{(t^{(n)} - t_r^k)^2}{2\sigma_p^2}\right), \qquad n = 1, 2, ..., N, \quad (4.37)$$

where t_r^k is a random variable with f_{t_r} distribution, that denotes the kth photon's registration time.

We aim to calculate the diagonal elements of the covariance matrix S_p :

$$
\begin{aligned}
S_p(n, n) &= E[(\tilde{y}(n) - y(n))^2], & (4.38)\\
&= E[(\tilde{y}(n) - E[\tilde{y}(n)] + E[\tilde{y}(n)] - y(n))^2] \\
&= E[(\tilde{y}(n) - E[\tilde{y}(n)])^2] + (E[\tilde{y}(n)] - y(n))^2 \\
&= \text{Var}(\tilde{y}(n)) + \text{Bias}^2(\tilde{y}(n)), & n = 1, 2, ..., N. \quad (4.39)
\end{aligned}
$$

According to the Eq. (4.36):

$$
\begin{aligned}
E[\tilde{y}(n)] &= N_p E[\tilde{y}_k(n)], & (4.40)\\
\text{Var}(\tilde{y}(n)) &= N_p \text{Var}(\tilde{y}_k(n)), & n = 1, 2, ..., N. \quad (4.41)
\end{aligned}
$$

Estimates of the $\text{Var}(\tilde{y}(n))$ and $\text{Bias}(\tilde{y}(n))$ were introduced in Refs. [81, 82]. Assuming that the underlying pdf function f_{t_r} is sufficiently smooth, and that $\sigma_p \to 0$ with $N_p\sigma_p \to \infty$ as $N_p \to \infty$, the Taylor series expansion gives:

$$\text{Bias}(\tilde{y}(n)) \approx \beta \frac{\sigma_p^2 f_{tr}''(t^{(n)})}{2}, \tag{4.42}$$

$$\text{Var}(\tilde{y}(n)) \approx \beta^2 \frac{f_{tr}(t^{(n)})}{2\sqrt{\pi} N_p \sigma_p}, \qquad n = 1, 2, ..., N, \tag{4.43}$$

where $f_{tr}''(t^{(n)})$ is a second derivative of the pdf function $f_{tr}(t^{(n)})$. Above approximations may be inaccurate for finite N_p, especially in the case discussed in this investigation, where the number of registered photo-electrons N_p is of the order of hundreds. Therefore, a new method to evaluate the $\text{Var}(\tilde{y}(n))$ and $\text{Bias}(\tilde{y}(n))$ for finite N_p was proposed. The method has been described in great details in the appendix A.2 and it was shown that the values of $\text{Var}(\tilde{y}), \text{Bias}(\tilde{y})$ may be estimated as:

$$\text{Bias}(\tilde{y}(n)) \approx \beta \left(\frac{2\Phi(t^{(n)}, \lambda\sigma_p)}{3\sqrt{2\pi}\sigma_p} - f_{tr}(t^{(n)}) \right), \tag{4.44}$$

$$\text{Var}(\tilde{y}(n)) \approx \beta^2 \frac{9\Phi(t^{(n)}, \lambda\sigma_p) + 8\Phi^2(t^{(n)}, \lambda\sigma_p) - 16\Phi^3(t^{(n)}, \lambda\sigma_p)}{36\pi N_p \sigma_p^2}, \tag{4.45}$$

for $n = 1, 2, ..., N$, where λ is the parameter defining the range of the second argument of function Φ:

$$\Phi(t^{(n)}, \lambda\sigma_p) = F_{tr}(t^{(n)} + \lambda\sigma_p) - F_{tr}(t^{(n)} - \lambda\sigma_p), \qquad n = 1, 2, ..., N, \tag{4.46}$$

and $F_{tr}(t^{(n)})$ is the cumulative distribution function of $f_{tr}(t^{(n)})$ calculated at $t^{(n)}$. Discussion of Eqs (4.44, 4.45) is given in the appendix A.2.

It should be underlined that both estimation methods, proposed (Eqs. (4.44, 4.45)) and based on Taylor series approximation (Eqs. (4.42, 4.43)), have the same asymptotic properties.[4] It may be shown that for $\sigma_p \to 0$ with $N_p\sigma_p \to \infty$ as $N_p \to \infty$:

$$\text{Bias}(\tilde{y}(n)) = 0,$$
$$\text{Var}(\tilde{y}(n)) = 0,$$

for $n = 1, 2, ..., N$.

4.4.2 Derivation of the coincidence resolving time

In the following we evaluate the CRT based on the standard deviation (σ_Θ) defined in Eq. (4.35). The lower limit of the CRT is defined by

---

[4] L. Raczyński et al., Calculation of the time resolution of the J-PET tomograph using kernel density estimation, *Phys. Med. Biol.* **62** (2017) 5083–5084.

the time spread due to the unknown depth-of-interaction (DOI) in a single scintillator. It should be stressed that this factor gains importance for large scintillator detectors, as in the J-PET for example. Since the interactions may occur with nearly equal probability along the whole thickness (D) of the plastic scintillator, time spread in a single scintillator may be well approximated by the uniform distribution with the width of D/c, where c denotes the γ photon speed. This implies that the distribution of the time difference between two detected γ photons has a triangle form with FWHM equal to D/c. The CRT may be estimated with the formula:

$$\text{CRT} = \sqrt{(2.35\sqrt{2})^2\sigma_\Theta^2 + \frac{D^2}{c^2}}, \tag{4.47}$$

where the first term describes the conversion of the standard deviation of distribution of interaction time in a single strip (σ_Θ) to the FWHM of annihilation event time uncertainty.[5]

---

[5] L. Raczyński et al., Calculation of the time resolution of the J-PET tomograph using kernel density estimation, *Phys. Med. Biol.* **62** (2017) 5082.

5. High-level data processing in Jagiellonian PET

This chapter describes the subsequent steps of high-level data processing in the J-PET scanner. The goal of high-level reconstruction is an estimation of radioactive tracer distribution injected to the patient's body. The image reconstruction is based on information on registered set of events of positron-electron annihilations. As it was discussed in the previous chapter, a single event is derived based on the detection of both γ photons in two scintillators in a narrow time window.

In recent years, PET data acquisition has been shifted to list-mode [10], where each registered event is saved individually. Storing coincidence events individually, instead of accumulated counts in sinogram, is preferred for efficient data processing for whole-body PET scanners that additionally record TOF information. Moreover, in list-mode data, each event may be described with additional information such as, e.g., deposited energy in the scintillators, detection time difference. Therefore, each event may be described with preselected set of features, creating high-dimensional feature space.

During the PET examination, an event is regarded as valid if: two γ photons are registered within a predefined time window, and the energy deposited in the scintillator by both γ photons exceeds the selected threshold. However, a number of events registered as having met the above criteria are undesirable. Different types of events in PET measurement are:

- *true*. Pair of γ photons derive from a single positron-electron annihilation and reach the scintillators without interacting with the atoms in detector volume.

- *random*. Pair of γ photons derive from two different positron-electron annihilations occur at approximately the same time.

- *scattered*. Pair of γ photons derive from a single positron-electron annihilation when one or both of them have undergone a Compton interaction.

As the true events are essential for the PET imaging, the random and scattered events distort the reconstructed distribution of radiotracer.

This chapter is organized as follows. First, in section 5.1, the method for classification of events will be proposed. For this purpose we apply a self-organizing map (SOM) network to analyse the high-dimensional feature space created by a set of three types of events. In particular, we provide a visualisation of high-dimensional feature space and we investigate the class distributions on a 2-dimensional SOM. Next, in section 5.2, we will introduce 3-dimensional, semi-analytic image reconstruction method. The key component of the proposed approach is the application of the Total Variation (TV) regularization in the image space during the analytic reconstruction filtering step, that is, after the TOF data have been TOF back-projected into the image space. The most important part of our investigations is the evaluation of the kernel operator, corresponding to the linear transform mapping an original radioactive tracer distribution into a TOF back-projected image. In section 5.2 the formula for calculations of the kernel operator will be introduced and proven.

5.1   Event classification in the J-PET detector

The are variety of methods for estimation of the contribution of random, scattered and true events during the PET examination. For instance, the fraction of random events may be estimated using a delayed coincidence window technique [83]. On the other hand, the contribution of scattered events may be evaluated using Single Scatter Simulation, in which scatter sinograms are simulated and appropriately scaled using the outside-of-body scatter tail [84,85]. Therefore, the purpose of this work is not related to the development of novel techniques for random and scattered events correction. Instead, we introduce the SOM network for visualisation of high-dimensional feature space of all types of registered events in 2-dimensional space. First, we present the set of selected features for visualization and classification purposes in section 5.1.1. Next, in section 5.1.2, we introduce a mathematical tool for assesement of quality of dimensionality reduction using SOM. Finally, in section 5.1.3, we present a simple event classication scheme using probabilistic approach.

5.1.1 Extraction of event features

We assume that each event is described by six features; thus it may be considered as a point in 6-dimensional (6-D) space. The first feature describes the angular distance in transaxial section between two scintillator strips that registered both γ photons in coincidence. The data are preliminary selected and only events with angular distance larger than 20° are further analysed. The second feature is the absolute value of registration time difference. The upper limit of time difference, i.e., coincidence time window, is set to 4 ns and is related to the size of the J-PET detector. The third feature describes the distance between the positions in the scintillators of two reconstructed γ photons. The fourth and fifth features store the information about the energy deposited by γ photons in both scintillator strips. In particular, the fourth feature defines the sum of energies and fifth feature defines the absolute value of difference of energies. The last feature, extracted based on attenuation map of the phantom, describes the attenuation coefficient along each LOR.

5.1.2 Dimensionality reduction using SOM

Consider a data set containing all three types of events reconstructed according to the low-level signal processing described in chapter 4. Each individual event is represented as a 6-D vector. The SOM is organized into a 2-D rectangular grid of size N_g (total number of neurons is N_g^2) and is trained using the set of 6-D input data. Once trained, the map can assign each event from the feature space to the neuron in the 2-D grid with the closest weight vector to the 6-D vector. However, it is highly likely that the input 6-D dataset is curved and cannot be mapped adequately on a 2-D plane, even using non-linear transit functions as in case of the SOM. Therefore, we propose a simple procedure for testing the quality of transformation of the 6-D feature space into 2-D grid. For this purpose we calculate the quantization error, denoted hereafter as q_e, for a trained SOM. q_e is defined as the mean value of Euclidean norms of the differences of all 6-D vectors describing event features in data set and the BMUs in the 2-D grid.

As other quantization techniques, the SOM allows to divide an input data set into groups, represented by their centroid point, i.e., node in the grid. Consider a SOM stacked in a 2-D rectangular grid, defined in the same way as described above, applied to the 2-D data set. Since the SOM model with fixed size (N_g) is optimized in order to minimize q_e, then for given data set we may postulate that:

$$q_e \cdot N_g = \text{const.} \tag{5.1}$$

Eq. (5.1) describes the fundamental property of the vector quantizations methods [86, 87]. It should be stressed that the relation in Eq. (5.1) is true for a given set, independently of the distribution of the original data in the 2-D space. This is because all the vectors are on the same 2-D plane. The specific distribution of the input 2-D vectors influence only on the constant value on the right hand side of Eq. (5.1).

In general the property introduced in Eq. (5.1) may be applied also to N-D data sets, where N > 2. The relation in Eq. (5.1) for N-D data holds only if the input N-D vectors may be fitted on non-linear 2-D surface. The main idea of learning process of the SOM neural network is to approximate the localization of this non-linear 2-D surface. The quality of this approximation may be evaluated based on the Eq. (5.1) as follow. We perform bilateral logarithm of the formula in Eq. (5.1):

$$\log(q_e \cdot N_g) = \xi,$$
$$\log(q_e) + \log(N_g) = \xi,$$
$$\log(q_e) = -\log(N_g) + \xi, \tag{5.2}$$

where ξ is a constant value. For a given N-D data set under investigation, we conduct numerous trainings of SOM networks with different number of neurons in the grid. For each network with N_g^2 neurons, a quantization error is evaluated. With all the collection of numbers N_g and corresponding errors q_e, the linear fit according to the formula

$$\log(q_e) = -\kappa \cdot \log(N_g) + \xi \tag{5.3}$$

is provided, in order to deliver parameters κ and ξ. As mentioned, ξ is related to the constant value in Eq. (5.2) and is not further analyzed. On the other hand, parameter κ describes the coplanarity of the input data, i.e., reflects the quality of approximation of the non-linear 2-D surface with SOM structure. From the comparison of Eq. (5.2) and Eq. (5.3) it is seen that $0 \leq \kappa \leq 1$. The value of κ close to 0 suggests very low dependence of the quantization error on the size of the SOM neural network; input N-D data set is not presented reliably by the map. However, the value close to 1 reflects very accuarate fit of the 2-D SOM grid on N-D space occupied by the analyzed data set.

5.1.3   Event classification using SOM

The trained SOM neural network with N_g^2 nodes allows to classify the events based on a simple probabilistic model. Consider that the probability than neuron (i, j) won is denoted as $\mathbb{P}(W_{ij})$, where $i, j = 1, \ldots, N_g$. The posterior pdf of the class c_k conditional on position i, j of the winning node on the map is denoted as

$$\mathbb{P}(c_k|W_{ij}) = \frac{\mathbb{P}(c_k \cap W_{ij})}{\mathbb{P}(W_{ij})} \quad k = 1, \ldots, N_c \tag{5.4}$$

where N_c stands for the number of event classes. Since

$$\mathbb{P}(W_{ij}) = \sum_{k=1}^{N_c} \mathbb{P}(c_k \cap W_{ij}) \tag{5.5}$$

we have

$$\sum_{k=1}^{N_c} \mathbb{P}(c_k|W_{ij}) = 1. \tag{5.6}$$

The proposed event classification procedure consists of two steps. First, for a new event, represented by a 6-D vector, the indexes (i, j) of the BMU in the SOM are evaluated. Next, the event is assigned to one of the classes $(k = 1, \ldots, N_c)$ that maximize the posterior pdf in Eq. (5.4), i.e.,

$$\hat{k} = \arg \max \mathbb{P}(c_k|W_{ij}).$$

Additionally, the SOM allows to predict the classifier performance by calculation of the information entropy. For a trained neural network, in each node i, j, the entropy may be calculated as follows:

$$E_{ij} = -\sum_{k=1}^{N_c} \mathbb{P}(c_k|W_{ij}) \cdot \log \mathbb{P}(c_k|W_{ij}). \tag{5.7}$$

Entropy E_{ij} takes minimal value equal to 0 when the probabilistic model described with conditional probability $\mathbb{P}(c_k|W_{ij})$ is determined, i.e., $\mathbb{P}(c_k|W_{ij}) = 1$ for one class and for all remaining classes it is 0. On the other hand, entropy E_{ij} is maximum when the conditional probability $\mathbb{P}(c_k|W_{ij})$ is the same for all classes, i.e., $\mathbb{P}(c_k|W_{ij}) = 1/N_c$ for $k = 1, \ldots, N_c$.

5.2   Image reconstruction using Total Variation regularization

Given good enough time resolution, a PET scanner using the TOF information could reconstruct each individual event with sufficient accuracy to measure the unknown radiotracer distribution directly. Currently however this is not the case and the measurements errors have to be incorporated into the reconstruction process. With the extra data dimension brought by TOF technique, typical registered TOF data are sparse in projection space; the dimensionality of the projection space is much higher than the number of TOF events. Therefore, processing of TOF data in projection space is unpractical, especially for the whole-body PET scanners and the most appropriate reconstruction techniques are list-mode (LM) approaches.

In this section we introduce a semi-analytic image reconstruction algorithm suited for the LM-TOF data structure. The recent results [88] suggest that as the CRT improves, the TOF analytic algorithms become more competitive to statistical iterative methods, e.g., TOF Maximum Likelihood Expectation Maximization (TOF-MLEM). In spite of the linear behavior and predictability, analytic methods exhibit higher sensitivity to the data noise, as compared to the statistical iterative approaches. This leads to more noisy images for low count data and thus affects the quantitative precision of the imaging studies. Consequently, proper regularization of the analytic reconstruction is of a very practical interest. The key component of the proposed method is the application of the TV regularization in the image space after the events have been TOF back-projected. Image space is substantially reduced in size as compared to the TOF data space, making the TV optimization operations much more efficient and practical. The procedure of the image reconstruction approach is as follows:

- *Data pre-correction.* As required for analytic reconstruction, in the first step LM-TOF events are pre-corrected. Pre-correction takes into account both the multiplicative factors (detector efficiency and attenuation factors) and the additive contamination of the data (random and scattered events). The latter issue was discussed in section 5.1.

- *TOF back-projection.* Corrected data are back-projected to the image space using the TOF information. The relation between the back-projected data and the unknown radiotracer distribution will be introduced in section 5.2.2.

- *Reconstruction with regularization.* The radiotracer distribution is reconstructed using the back-projected image by solving the unconstrained TV regularization problem. The reconstruction problem based on TV approach will be discussed in section 5.2.3.

The proposed algorithm is similar to the conventional back-projection filter (BPF) method [89]. However, in the BPF algorithm acquired data are first deposited into projection space. In contrast, in this approach the incorporation of the TOF information allows for direct transformation into the TOF back-projected image. Moreover, in the proposed work, the TV regularization acts as a filtering step, while in standard BPF or TOF-BPF algorithms, regularization is provided via apodizing functions. In the following sections we describe the subsequent steps of the proposed image reconstruction. We start with introduction of basic definitions and notation.

5.2.1 Background and notation

The 3-D TOF-PET data can be expressed as [90, 91]:

$$p(s, \phi, z_c, \theta, l) = \int_{-\infty}^{\infty} dl' f(\overrightarrow{x} = l'\overrightarrow{\omega_1} + s\overrightarrow{\omega_2} + z_c\overrightarrow{\omega_3})h(l - l') \qquad (5.8)$$

where the function $f(\overrightarrow{x} \triangleq (x, y, z))$ describes the radioactive tracer distribution, s and ϕ are the transaxial sinogram coordinates, z_c is the axial coordinate of the mid-point of the LOR, θ is the co-polar angle between the LOR and transaxial plane, l is the TOF variable and h is the TOF profile (see Fig. 5.1). Three unit vectors are defined as:

$$\overrightarrow{\omega_1} = (-\cos\theta\sin\phi, \cos\theta\cos\phi, \sin\theta) \qquad (5.9)$$
$$\overrightarrow{\omega_2} = (\cos\phi, \sin\phi, 0) \qquad (5.10)$$
$$\overrightarrow{\omega_3} = (0, 0, 1). \qquad (5.11)$$

The TOF profile h is often modeled as a Gaussian function [92] with standard deviation $\sigma = c \cdot \mathrm{CRT}/(4\sqrt{2\log 2})$, where c denotes the speed of light. The TOF variable l is related with the TOF time difference Δt between the two arrival times of the two photons by $l = c\Delta t/2$, where $l = 0$ corresponds to the position of the LOR mid-point.

An image is represented by a 3-D function $f(\overrightarrow{x})$, where $\overrightarrow{x} \in \mathbb{R}^3$ denotes the space coordinate. Discretized version of continuous function $f(x, y, z)$ is represented by f_{ijk}, where $(i, j, k) = 1, ..., n$ corresponds to

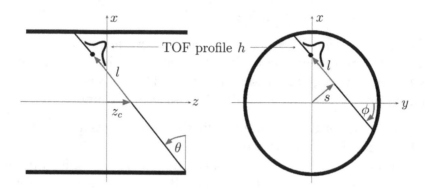

Figure 5.1. Schematic view of a cylindrical 3-D PET tomograph in axial cross-section (left panel) and transaxial cross-section (right panel).

the voxels position in the image matrix. The bold symbol $\mathbf{f} \in \mathbb{R}^N$, where $N = n^3$, represents the vectorized version of the matrix f. In general $n \times n \times n$ size images are stored as N length vectors.

The geometrical arrangement of discrete detectors in a scanner determines a set of samples $(s, \phi, z_c, \theta, l) \triangleq \vec{\Sigma} \in \mathbb{R}^5$ in the projection space. The most common arrangement is a ring scanner: an even number of detectors uniformly spaced along a circle and

$$\vec{\Sigma} = \{(s, \phi, z_c, \theta, l) : |s| \leq R_d, 0 \leq \phi \leq \pi,$$

$$|z_c| \leq \frac{L_d}{2}, 0 \leq \theta \leq \frac{\pi}{2}, |l| \leq \sqrt{R_d^2 + \frac{L_d^2}{4}}\},$$

where R_d is the detector radius, L_d is the detector length. Discretized TOF projection data are represented by the matrix element p_{ijkmq}, where (i, j, k, m, q) correspond to the variables $(s, \phi, z_c, \theta, l)$, respectively. The bold symbol $\mathbf{p} \in \mathbb{R}^P$, represents the vectorized version of the matrix p.

The mathematical operator mapping a function $f(\vec{x})$ into $p(\vec{\Sigma})$, according to Eq. (5.8), is denoted by $\mathcal{K}$:

$$p(\vec{\Sigma}) = (\mathcal{K}f)(\vec{\Sigma}) \tag{5.12}$$

and $K \in \mathbb{R}^{P \times N}$ is a finite-dimensional sampling of the $\mathcal{K}$ transform:

$$\mathbf{p} = K\mathbf{f} \tag{5.13}$$

and is often called a system matrix.

5.2.2 TOF convolution operator

As mentioned at the beginning of this section, the acquired set of events is deposited directly into TOF back-projected image. In the following we derive the relation between the TOF back-projected image and the original radioactive tracer distribution. We define a TOF back-projection operator ($\mathcal{K}^{\#}$) and we provide a linear transform of the projection data p defined in Eq. (5.12):

$$(\mathcal{K}^{\#}p)(\vec{x}) = (\mathcal{K}^{\#}\mathcal{K}f)(\vec{x}) \tag{5.14}$$

$$b(\vec{x}) = (\mathcal{K}^{\#}\mathcal{K}f)(\vec{x}) \tag{5.15}$$

$$b(\vec{x}) = \mathcal{A}f(\vec{x}) \tag{5.16}$$

where $\mathcal{A} = \mathcal{K}^{\#}\mathcal{K}$ is an overall TOF forward and back-projection operator and b is TOF back-projected image. The images f and b have the same sizes and one-to-one voxel correspondence. Under the assumption that the TOF profile h is shift invariant, so that the integral in Eq. (5.8) is a convolution, the operator $\mathcal{A}$ may be described as a convolution operator with a kernel $a(\vec{x})$:

$$b(\vec{x}) = a(\vec{x}) * f(\vec{x}). \tag{5.17}$$

The aspect of the validity of the kernel a shift-invariance assumption will be discussed in the last part of this section.

The kernel $a(\vec{x})$ may be easily derived for a point source $\delta(\vec{x})$ placed in the tomograph center based on Eq. (5.15), i.e.,

$$a(\vec{x}) = (\mathcal{K}^{\#}\mathcal{K}\delta)(\vec{x}). \tag{5.18}$$

In the following, by convention we use subscripts o to denote exact values as opposite to estimated quantities described with subscripts e. A measured TOF event is defined as a set $\vec{g_e} = (x_{u,e}, y_{u,e}, z_{u,e}, t_{u,e}, x_{d,e}, y_{d,e}, z_{d,e}, t_{d,e})$. The $(x_{u,e}, y_{u,e}, z_{u,e})$ and $(x_{d,e}, y_{d,e}, z_{d,e})$ denote the reconstructed position along the upper and lower strips, respectively, see Fig. 5.2 for details. The $t_{u,e}$ and $t_{d,e}$ are reconstructed hit times, such that:

$$l_e = c\frac{t_{d,e} - t_{u,e}}{2}. \tag{5.19}$$

An annihilation occurring at $\vec{x_o} = (0,0,0)$ is measured as the point $\vec{x_e} = \vec{x_o} + \vec{\epsilon}$, where

$$\vec{\epsilon} = l_e\vec{\omega}_{1,e} + s_e\vec{\omega}_{2,e} + z_{c,e}\vec{\omega}_3 \tag{5.20}$$

$$= \vec{\epsilon_1} + \vec{\epsilon_2} + \vec{\epsilon_3} \tag{5.21}$$

based on the parametrization introduced in Eq. (5.8). As it is shown in Fig. 5.2, the measurement error $\vec{\epsilon}$ is a vector with a component $\vec{\epsilon_1}$ describing TOF uncertainty, with a component $\vec{\epsilon_2}$ related to the unknown DOI in a single scintillator and with a component $\vec{\epsilon_3}$ describing uncertainty along axial direction (note that $\vec{\omega}_3$ is constant (see Eq. (5.11)) and therefore we do not use the subscripts). From Eq. (5.20) it may be seen that the measurement error $\vec{\epsilon}$ is evaluated after TOF back-projection of the TOF event $\vec{g_e}$ into the image space. Hence, assuming that the $\vec{\epsilon}$ is independent of the locations and measurement errors of all other annihilations, the $\vec{\epsilon}$ may be considered as a random variable with pdf given by the overall TOF forward and back-projection operator a in Eq. (5.18).

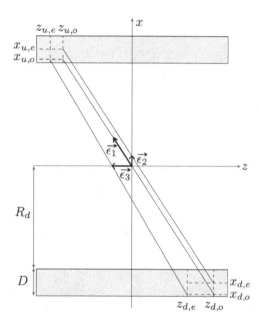

Figure 5.2.   Example of reconstruction of point source placed in the detector center presented in axial cross-section. The measurement error consists of three components: the TOF uncertainty, the unknown DOI, and the uncertainty along the axial direction.

The proposed mathematical model of measurement errors is inspired by the work of [93, 94]. In [93], the authors assumed that $\vec{\epsilon}$ is normally distributed and has two components: parallel and transverse to the LOR. The parallel component error is analogous to $\vec{\epsilon_1}$ in our derivation (see Fig. 5.2). However, instead of one transverse component error we considered two error vectors $\vec{\epsilon_2}, \vec{\epsilon_3}$ according to the parametrization given in Eq. (5.8). This approach allows us to include more information about geometrical arrangement and readout specification of different PET systems, e.g., the J-PET scanner, in our calculations.

In order to simplify further calculations, the following assumption is proposed. Note that in the most interesting case for large detector radius R_d, orientation of component error $\vec{\epsilon_1}$, i.e., vector $\vec{\omega}_{1,e}$ in Eq. (5.20), is very close to the true LOR direction $\vec{\omega}_{1,o}$. Therefore, we assume that $\vec{\epsilon_1} \approx l_e \vec{\omega}_{1,o}$, (see Fig. 5.2 for details) where only l_e is a random variable. Furthermore, the $\vec{\epsilon_2}$ and $\vec{\epsilon_3}$ in Eq. (5.20) depend only on transaxial $(x_{u,e}, y_{u,e}, x_{d,e}, y_{d,e})$ and axial $(z_{u,e}, z_{d,e})$ uncertainties, respectively. Hence, the error $\vec{\epsilon}$ may be approximated as a sum of three independent random variables and the unknown kernel a is given as the convolution:

$$a(\vec{x}) = \left(a_{(1)} * a_{(2)} * a_{(3)} \right)(\vec{x}) \tag{5.22}$$

where $a_{(k)}$ describes pdf of error term $\vec{\epsilon_k}$ in Eq. (5.20) for $k = 1, 2, 3$. It is shown in appendix A.3, that

$$a_{(1)}(\vec{x}) = \kappa_1 \frac{h(\|\vec{x}\|)\mathcal{C}(\vec{x}, \theta_{\mathrm{acc}})}{\|\vec{x}\|\sqrt{x^2 + y^2}} \tag{5.23}$$

$$a_{(2)}(\vec{x}) = \kappa_2 \frac{h_2(\sqrt{x^2 + y^2})}{\sqrt{x^2 + y^2}} \tag{5.24}$$

$$a_{(3)}(\vec{x}) = \frac{1}{\sqrt{\pi}\sigma_z} \exp\left(-\frac{z}{\sigma_z^2}\right). \tag{5.25}$$

The parameter θ_{acc} corresponds to the maximal accepted θ angle, κ_1, κ_2 stand for the normalization constants, h_2 is the profile function given in Eq. (A.15), function $\mathcal{C}$ is defined in Eq. (A.13), and σ_z is standard deviation of Gaussian function describing uncertainty of the measurement along axial position. It should be stressed that the kernel a does not have a finite support due to the Gaussian functions in $a_{(1)}$ and $a_{(3)}$. In order to reduce the reconstruction time, we assessed the truncation of the kernel a and this aspect will be investigated in section 6.6.1.

In the last part of this section, we discuss the validity of the kernel a shift-invariance assumption (see Eq. (5.17)). For this purpose we consider the influence of the position of point source on the distributions $a_{(k)}$ of measurement errors $\vec{\epsilon_k}$ for $k = 1, 2, 3$. The pdf $a_{(3)}$ does not depend on the position of point source as the uncertainty of measurement along the axial direction (z) is assumed to be constant (see appendix A.3.3 for details). The pdf $a_{(2)}$ for central and shifted point sources is not stationary since the efficient DOI changes with different angle in (x, y) cross-section between two detectors in coincidence. Under the assumption that annihilation photons propagate isotropically, only for central point source the angular difference in (x, y) cross-section between two detectors is always $\approx 180°$ (see appendix A.3.2 for details). However, kernel $a_{(2)}$ contributes only to the (x, y) distribution of the overall kernel a and as the TOF uncertainty is still a major challenge of current PET scanners, the investigation of influence of pdf $a_{(1)}$ on shift-invariance is of main importance. The main parameter that governs the distribution of kernel $a_{(1)}$ is θ_{acc} angle. Note that the θ_{acc} angle cannot be greater than maximum detection angle θ_{max} for the point source placed in the tomograph center:

$$\theta_{\text{max}} = \arctan\left(\frac{L_d}{2R_d}\right). \tag{5.26}$$

The solid angle covered by the tomograph is largest in the center (θ_{max}), but it decreases if one moves the point source from the center towards the edge. Consequently, the function describing the kernel a depends on the spatial location of the point source and is said to be spatially variant.

In the 1980s several 3-D analytic reconstruction approaches have been proposed to circumvent the assumption of shift-invariance [95, 96]. This has been done by completion of the missing regions by forward-projecting (re-projecting) images initially reconstructed from the subset of projection data for which $\theta \leq \theta_{\text{min}}$. The limiting angle θ_{min} imposes shift-invariance everywhere within the field of view specified by the volume of the reconstructed object.

In this work no initial image reconstruction and data re-projection was performed, and the shift-invariance was approximated by rejecting any events with $\theta \geq \theta_{\text{acc}}$, where $\theta_{\text{min}} \leq \theta_{\text{acc}} \leq \theta_{\text{max}}$. Increasing θ_{acc} weakens the assumption of shift-invariance of the kernel a, however, on the other hand ensures higher statistics. A trade-off between the number of accepted events and the size of the area inside the tomograph for which the shift-invariance assumption of kernel a holds is optimized by changing the θ_{acc} parameter.

It is worth noting that the detection angle limitation is required in case of long PET detectors. A more oblique LOR penetrates more scintillating material than a LOR of less axial difference, which coupled with unknown depth of interaction degrades the axial resolution. For instance, for a 200 cm long EXPLORER scanner [41, 42], the maximum axial difference between crystal pairs was limited to 115 cm. Moreover, the restriction on maximal θ angle is beneficial due to the photons attenuation effect in the patient's body; the more oblique the LOR the longer the path through the patient's body and higher the probability of photon attenuation.

5.2.3 TOF reconstruction with TV regularization

The problem in Eq. (5.17) may be rewritten to the matrix notation:

$$\mathbf{b} = A\mathbf{f} \tag{5.27}$$

where A is finite-dimensional sampling of operator $\mathcal{A}$ and therefore has a circulant structure (see Eqs (5.16)-(5.17) for details). The circulant property of matrix A is a critical factor to speed up the algorithm as it allows the use of Fourier transform methods.

Since the TOF back-projected image $\mathbf{b}$ is not a perfect noiseless image, the inverse problem defined in Eq. (5.27) is ill-posed and the application of some regularization technique is required. The most common class of regularization methods in image processing is based on TV approach. Brief description and discussion of the TV-norm of 3-D images is provided in section 3.2.

Optimization algorithm finds a solution $\hat{\mathbf{f}}$ of Eq. (5.27) by solving an unconstrained regularization problem:

$$\hat{\mathbf{f}} = \arg\min \quad TV(\mathbf{f}) + \frac{\mu}{2}\|A\mathbf{f} - \mathbf{b}\|_2^2, \tag{5.28}$$

which is known as the TV/L2 minimization. The μ is the regularization parameter. The data fidelity term in Eq. (5.28) is a L2 norm that constitutes the Gaussian noise model. Note that the image $\mathbf{b}$ is evaluated after the pre-correction of the data, which are no longer described by the Poisson distribution and it is convenient to assume the Gaussian noise model. The theory of penalty functions implies that the solution of Eq. (5.28) approaches the solution of Eq. (5.27) as μ goes to infinity. The proposed algorithm is based on the augmented Lagrangian method [60, 61] and is presented in details in section 3.2. This algorithm will be denoted hereafter as TOF-BPTV (TOF Back Projection Total Variation regularization).

PET reconstruction using TV regularization was investigated by several groups. The approach proposed in this dissertation is inspired by a regularization procedure for PET first introduced in [97]. Given a noisy projection data $\mathbf{p}$, an image is reconstructed by solving:

$$\min_{\mathbf{f}} \quad \alpha_0 TV(K\mathbf{f}) + \alpha_1\|\mathbf{f}\|_1 + \frac{\alpha_2}{2}\|K\mathbf{f} - \mathbf{p}\|_2^2 \tag{5.29}$$

where $\alpha_0, \alpha_1, \alpha_2$ are positive parameters. In this method TV regularization acts only on the $K\mathbf{f}$. As an extension, in [98] an image from PET measurements has been reconstructed by smoothing both in projection and in image space:

$$\min_{\mathbf{f}} \quad \alpha_0 \, \mathrm{TV}(K\mathbf{f}) + \alpha_1 \, \mathrm{TV}(\mathbf{f}) + \sum_i \frac{(K_i \mathbf{f} - \mathbf{p}_i)^2}{\mathbf{p}_i} \tag{5.30}$$

where α_0, α_1 are positive parameters.

In both methods, the reconstruction problem does not include the 3-D image space and TOF information. Instead, 2-D image space and non TOF data are considered, which results in 2-D projection space p. Consideration of additional dimensions increases significantly the size of the system matrix K making the optimization problems in Eqs (5.29)−(5.30) invariably large-scale. In fact, in that case storing the full 5-D system matrix in memory is impossible, even in sparse format. Moreover, the matrix K does not have a circulant structure as the matrix A in Eq. (5.28).

This implies that these methods could not be used as the reference to the proposed technique. On the other hand, almost every current PET image reconstruction algorithm is based on likelihood maximization approach [99, 100]. Therefore as the reference method, TOF-MLEM algorithm has been selected. Moreover, we will provide the comparative studies with TOF-FBP algorithm, in order to investigate the computational speed of the proposed approach.

6. Results

6.1 Experimental and simulation scenarios

For the evaluation of the proposed data processing algorithms described in chapters 4 and 5, both experimental and simulation data of the J-PET scanner were used. The performance of the low-level signal processing methods, presented in chapter 4, is investigated by using a data set of reference signals registered in a single module scintillator strip of the J-PET detector. This experimental setup is described in section 6.1.1. The quality of the high-level data processing methods, introduced in chapter 5, is examined by using both experimental and simulation data. The experimental scenario describing the 3-layer prototype J-PET scanner is shown in section 6.1.2 and the simulated 1-layer J-PET detector is introduced in section 6.1.3.

6.1.1 Experimental scheme with 1 scintillator strip

In this section we introduce the scheme with single detection module of J-PET device that allows the investigation of low-level data processing described in chapter 4. The scheme of the experimental setup is presented in Fig. 6.1.

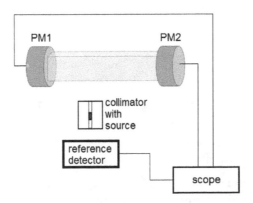

Figure 6.1. Scheme of the experimental setup with single detection module.

The single detection module is built from the BC-420 plastic scintillator strip, with dimensions of $5 \times 19 \times 300$ mm, readout at two ends by Hamamatsu R4998 photomultipliers is denoted as PM1(2). Measurements are performed using γ photon from a ^{22}Na source placed inside the lead collimator between the scintillator strip and the reference detector. The reference detector consists of a small scintillator strip with a thickness of 4 mm. A collimated beam emerging through a slit 1.5 mm wide and 20 cm long is used for irradiating desired points across the strip. In order to detect the event, coincident registration of signals from the PM1 and a reference detector is required. Such trigger conditions reduce the background from the deexcitation photon (1.27 MeV) to a negligible level [17]. The time of triggering by the reference detector is used to estimate the event arrival time. The constant electronic time delay between the true event time and the measured time of arrival at the reference detector does not influence the time and spatial resolutions and is shifted to zero. The full waveforms of signals on PM1 and PM2 are sampled using the Lecroy SDA 6000A oscilloscope with a sampling interval of 50 ps.

The ^{22}Na source is moved along the line parallel to the scintillator strip from the first to the second end in steps of 6 mm. At each position, about 5000 pairs of signals from PM1 and PM2 are registered in coincidence. The length of registered signals, denoted as $\tilde{y}$ according to the description in section 4.4.1, is set to 15 ns, which corresponds to $N = 300$ samples. Since the absolute registration time has no physical meaning, we synchronize the signals in data set in such way that the fixed index number 20 corresponds to the amplitude of 0.06 V on the rising slope of each signal. An example of a signal registered at PM1 is presented in Fig. 6.2.

6.1.2 The prototype J-PET scanner with 192 scintillator strips

This section describes the J-PET scanner prototype, which is the first 3D TOF-PET scanner built of plastic scintillators having axially arranged strips forming a cylindrical diagnostic chamber. The detector constructed at the Jagiellonian University is composed of 192 modules based on strips of EJ-230 plastic scintillator, arranged into a barrel with 3-layers (see Fig. 6.3). The inner and the middle layers are composed of 48 modules, whereas the third (outer) layer consists of 96 modules. Layers do not directly overlay each other and are 85 cm, 93.5 cm and 115 cm in

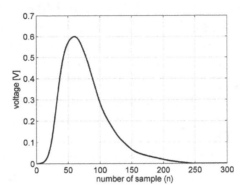

Figure 6.2. Signal observed in the photomultiplier output generated by interaction in the center of the scintillator strip (the meaning of variable n is the same as in Eq. (4.8)).

diameter, respectively. Each scintillator strip is 50 cm long with a rectangular cross section of 0.7×1.9 cm^2. Within a detection module, both ends of the scintillator strip are optically coupled to Hamamatsu R9800 photomultipliers.

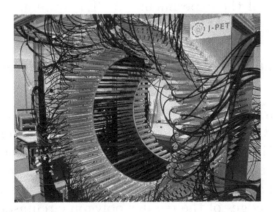

Figure 6.3. A photo of the J-PET detector consisting of 192 plastic scintillator strips arranged in 3 concentric layers.

Experiments with J-PET prototype were performed with six point-like sources of ^{22}Na placed in positions suggested by the National Electrical Manufacturers Association (NEMA) in the NEMA-NU-2-2012 norm [101]. While in the norm it is suggested to measure the source subsequently in each position, in our study six point-like sources were measured at the same time. Sources were placed at the following positions: $(x, y, z) =$ (0 cm, 1 cm, 0 cm), (0 cm, 10 cm, 0 cm), (0 cm, 20 cm, 0 cm), (0 cm,

1 cm, -18.75 cm), (0 cm, 10 cm, -18.75 cm) and (0 cm, 20 cm, -18.75 cm). A dedicated styrofoam panel was prepared for measurements; the sources were attached to the panel using adhesive tape. Styrofoam was chosen because of its low density and small probability for scattering and attenuation on the panel.

A coincident event is defined as a set of consecutive interactions of photons, originating from a single annihilation and all interactions of secondary particles. The interactions are considered to originate from the same coincident event if they are detected within the fixed time window of 4 ns. This number ensures that the probability that interactions from two different events are ascribed to the same event is below 1 permille. Based on our previous studies [17, 102], only the events with exactly two interactions registered with an energy loss above the 200 keV threshold each are accepted. For the study with six point-like sources, a total of 70 million coincident events, fullfiling the above energy condition, are recorded.

As was shown in [20], the resulting time resolution (CRT) of the 3-layer prototype J-PET scanner is about 500 ps. The corresponding axial spatial resolution of the experimental J-PET system, i.e., FWHM along the z coordinate, is equal to about 4.5 cm.

6.1.3   The simulated J-PET scanner with 384 scintillator strips

In the last scenario, the ideal geometry of the J-PET detector was simulated with the Geant4 application for tomographic emission (GATE) software [103, 104]. The simulated scanner is composed of axially oriented scintillator strips, arranged into a barrel with 1-layer with an inner radius of 42.8 cm and length of 50 cm. The number of strips is calculated as the number of edges of the regular polygon circumscribed around the ring with the radius 42.8 cm and equals 384 (see Fig. 6.4). Each scintillator strip is assumed to have the same physical properties and dimensions as the prototype scanner, i.e., is made of BC-420 material and has a rectangular cross section of 0.7×1.9 cm^2.

The simulations with single layer J-PET detector were performed with the NEMA IEC body phantom (see Fig. 6.4). The phantom includes six spheres and one long cylinder, and is simulated according to the specification given in [101]. The four smallest spheres of 10, 13, 17 and 22 mm diameter simulate hot lesions with contrast ratio of 4 : 1, with respect to the activity concentration of the background. The two largest spheres of

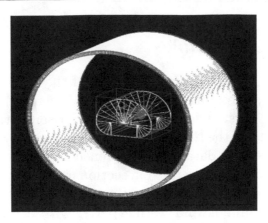

Figure 6.4.   Schematic view of the one layer J-PET detector consisting of 384 plastic scintillator strips with NEMA IEC body phantom inside. The figure was generated in GATE software [103, 104].

28 and 37 mm diameter simulate cold lesions with no radioactivity. The centers of all six spheres are in the same transaxial plane and located at 7 cm from the phantom lid. The 18 cm long cold cylinder of 51 mm diameter is inserted on the central axis of the phantom. We model an injected activity of 53 MBq of ^{18}F-FDG dissolved in water.

For the NEMA IEC phantom simulation, a total of 50.0 million coincident events are recorded, corresponding approximately to a twenty-minute scan for a real J-PET acquisition. The total number of events includes 20.0 million trues, 9.4 million scatters and 20.6 million randoms. Each coincidence fulfills the same conditions as in the case of experiments with the J-PET prototype described in section 6.1.2; the coincidence is stored only if two interactions with an energy loss above the 200 keV threshold are captured within the time window of 4 ns.

As the MC simulation does not take into account the spatial and time measurement uncertainties, an additional smearing using experimental resolutions of the detector was applied. The CRT and axial spatial resolution are simulated for SiPM readout solution of the J-PET scanner. The values of CRT and FWHM in the z coordinate for SiPMs were estimated based on simulations presented in [19] and are equal to 230 ps and 2 cm, respectively.

6.2 Recovery of signal waveform based on limited number of samples

In this section, we demonstrate the results of the recovery of full signals waveform on the photomultplier output based on few samples. We show that the number of samples (M) required to sense the signal can be considerably less than the total number of time samples (N). The method is validated by using a data set of reference signals registered in single module scintillator strip, described in section 6.1.2, of the J-PET scanner.

The complete data set of reference signals (Y) was divided into two disjoint subsets: training and testing parts, with a ratio of 9 : 1. The training data set Y was transformed via PCA into a new space X according to the Eq. (4.15). The evaluated matrix A was saved and used in the further analysis during the signal x recovery, see Eq. (4.16) for details. In order to find the theoretical value of mean recovery error σ_x^2 as a function of the number of samples M, one needs to specify the following parameters: σ, D, τ (see Eq. (4.20) for details). The standard deviation of the noise (σ) was estimated based on the training data set Y to ca. 0.015 V, which is consistent with the oscilloscope specification. The unknown parameters D, τ were found after the analysis of diagonal elements of the covariance matrix P of the training data set X. The smallest value D and the largest value τ for which the condition from Eq. (4.19) was met, are equal to 4.2 V^2 and 0.33, respectively.

It should be stressed that, for a given number of samples (M), the expected value of σ_x^2 in J-PET scenario would be slightly greater than for the one described by Eq. (4.20). The reason is that the signals are probed in the voltage domain and hence in the case when the amplitude of the signal is smaller than the threshold level, not all the samples of the signal are acquired. In other words, the effective number of samples varies from measurement to measurement and is always less than or equal to M. Therefore, in order to evaluate the theoretical function of mean recovery error in the J-PET scenario, both the values of the threshold levels and the distribution of signal amplitides have to be specified first. The experimental cumulative distribution function (cdf), based on the signals registered at all the positions along the scintillator strip, is presented in Fig. 6.5. The amplitudes of the signals are in the range from 0.3 V to 1.0 V. The signals with amplitude smaller than a 0.3 V are filtered out due to the requirement on the minimal energy deposition, i.e., 200 keV. Hence, a sharp edge on cdf for this value is observed in Fig. 6.5.

We simulate a front-end electronic device that probes the signals at

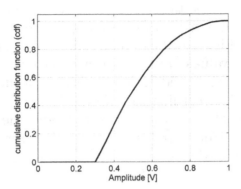

Figure 6.5. Experimental cumulative distribution function of signal amplitudes.

preselected number of voltage levels, both on the rising and falling slopes, based on the fully sampled signals stored in testing data set Y. We carry out the experiments for different numbers of voltage levels from 2 to 15. In each case, the level of 0.06 V on the rising slope is used for triggering purposes and is common for all signals, as was mentioned in section 6.1.1. Therefore, the effective number of simulated samples (M) is equal to the total number of samples on the rising and falling slopes minus one. In particular, for the measurement with four-levels, which is of most importance since the currently developed front-end electronic allows one to probe the signals at four fixed-voltage levels, $M = 7$. The remaining thresholds are adjusted after a simple optimization process, where the goal is to minimize the experimental mean recovery error σ_x^2. In case of the J-PET electronics, the optimal values of the four voltage levels are: 0.06, 0.20, 0.35 and 0.60 V.

For a fixed number (M) and voltage levels, signal recovery is provided bellow. The samples at optimal thresholds are selected to simulate the measurement y_Ω based on fully sampled waveforms of signals from testing data set Y. The measurement matrix A_Ω is formed from the selected rows of matrix A. Next, the signal $\hat{x}$ is recovered using Eq. (4.16), and finally the signal $\hat{y}$ is derived.

Since the amplitude of the signal may be less than certain voltage levels, not all samples had to be acquired, i.e. the number of samples is $\leq M$. In particular, for optimal values of four voltage thresholds $(M = 7)$, only for about 30% of signals, amplitudes are greater than 0.60 V, and all samples are available; the experimental cdf of amplitudes of the signals, presented in Fig. 6.5, takes the value 0.7 for the highest voltage level. According to the theoretical calculations only for this fraction of signals, the average recovery error takes the smallest value $\sigma_x^2(7) \approx 0.173$ V^2. Moreover, for about 55% of signals with amplitudes between 0.35 V and 0.60 V according to Fig. 6.5, the effective number of samples is equal to 5 and the theoretical value of average recovery error is $\sigma_x^2(5) \approx 0.228$ V^2. For the rest of the considered signals, with amplitudes below 0.35 V (about 15% of signals according to cdf distribution shown in Fig. 6.5), the effective number of samples is equal to 3 and the theoretical value of average recovery error is $\sigma_x^2(3) \approx 0.346$ V^2. Finally, the effective theoretical mean value of recovery error in the J-PET scenario for four voltage levels is:

$$\sigma_{x(\text{eff})}^2(7) \approx 30\% \cdot \sigma_x^2(7) + 55\% \cdot \sigma_x^2(5) + 15\% \cdot \sigma_x^2(3)$$
$$\approx 30\% \cdot 0.173 + 55\% \cdot 0.228 + 15\% \cdot 0.346$$
$$\approx 0.229 \text{ V}^2$$

and is higher than the theoretical value for $M = 7$ samples.

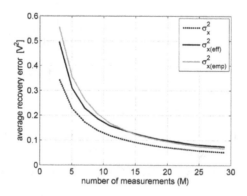

Figure 6.6. Comparison of average recovery errors σ_x^2 as a function of the acquired samples (M). Meaning of the curves is described in the text.

Evaluated theoretical and experimental curves describing the average recovery error as a function of the number of samples (M) in the J-PET experiment are shown in Fig. 6.6. An empirical mean value of $\sigma_{x(\text{emp})}^2$ is marked with a solid gray line in Fig. 6.6 and is very similar to the effective, theoretical characteristic ($\sigma_{x(\text{eff})}^2$) marked with a solid black line, that takes into account the distribution of amplitudes presented in Fig. 6.5. The difference between those two functions is larger for small values of M (about 10% of absolute value) and almost negligible for greater numbers of samples. As explained before, both of these functions differ significantly from the theoretical characteristic of σ_x^2, calculated according to

Eq. (4.20), marked with dashed black line in Fig. 6.6.

The analysis of the characteristic of average recovery error allows us to indicate the required number of samples to signal recovery. The function $\sigma_x^2(M)$ is approximately proportional to $1/M$ but, due to the logarithmic factor (see Eq.(4.20)), it drops rapidly until M reaches the value of about 10. Further increase in the number of samples does not provide any significant improvement in the signal recovery. This is very important information, since the currently developed front-end electronic provides eight time values for each signal ($M = 7$).

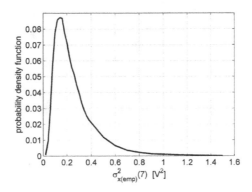

Figure 6.7. Probability density function of the experimental recovery error evaluated for four voltage levels ($\sigma_{x(\text{emp})}^2(7)$).

The probability density function of the recovery error $||x^0 - \hat{x}||_2^2$ evaluated using all signals from the testing data set for four voltage levels 0.06, 0.20, 0.35 and 0.60 V is shown in Fig. 6.7. From the experimental distribution of $||x^0 - \hat{x}||_2^2$ one may observe that the recovery error is concentrated between 0 and 0.4 V^2 with the tail reaching the value 1.5 V^2. As it was shown in Fig. 6.6, the average $\sigma_{x(\text{emp})}^2(7)$ is about 0.264 V^2. The median of a probability distribution of a recovery error is equal to ca. 0.192 V^2.

Two signal recovery examples, with medium and large recovery error, are shown in Fig. 6.8 and 6.9, respectively. The values of the signal recovery errors in Fig. 6.8 and 6.9 are 0.266 and 0.814 V^2. As expected, the worst situation occurs when the amplitude of the signal is slightly below the threshold level (see Fig. 6.9) or when it is much larger than the highest voltage threshold. In our sampling scheme the highest recovery errors are observed for signals with amplitude in the range from 0.55 to 0.6 V and from 0.95 to 1 V (where 1 V corresponds to the maximum amplitude, see Fig. 6.5). Unfortunately, there is no possibility to overcome these phenomena when only a few samples of the signal are available. On the other hand, it can be seen that the average recovery error is on an acceptable level. In a typical situation the signal is recovered quite accurately (see Fig. 6.8).

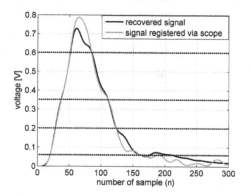

Figure 6.8. Example of signal recovery based on samples registered on four voltage levels; the recovery error is about 0.266 V^2.

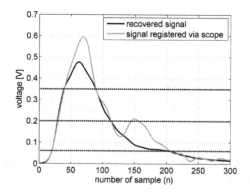

Figure 6.9. Example of signal recovery based on samples registered on four voltage levels; the recovery error is about 0.814 V^2. Since the amplitude of the signal is smaller than 0.6 V, samples from highest level are unavailable.

6.3   Reconstruction of γ photon interaction position in scintillator

In the J-PET scanner a position of γ photon interaction along the scintillator strip is reconstructed based on the measurement of times of light signals arrival to photomultipliers. In this section, we investigate the method for hit-position reconstruction, described in section 4.3, in order to evaluate a spatial resolution of the J-PET detector. As described in previous section 6.2, we simulate a four-level measurement based on the training data set of fully sampled signals acquired with the single detection module (see Fig. 6.1). We perform the analysis for both types of the input data, raw samples registered on four voltage levels (8 samples per signal) and of the fully recovered waveforms (300 samples per signal).

6.3.1   Hit-position reconstruction using raw samples

In the first step, we investigate the spatial resolution obtained from the original raw samples. As mentioned in section 6.2, the optimal values of the four voltage levels are: 0.06, 0.20, 0.35 and 0.60 V. The effective number of acquired variables is smaller by one and equal to 15, since only differences of times are physically meaningful. Therefore, each single measurement is represented by a 15-dimensional real number vector.

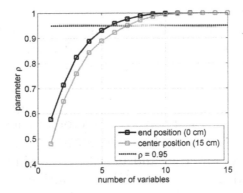

Figure 6.10. Explained variance (parameter ρ) as a function of the assumed number of independent variables. The horizontal line indicates the criterion for the determination of the minimum number of degrees of freedom.

In order to estimate the number of effective degrees of freedom in each dataset, the PCA is performed and subsequently the parameter ρ, describing an explained variance, is determined as a function of the number of variables. Details of the procedure were presented in section 4.3. Two curves representing signals registered in two most peripheral places are shown in Fig. 6.10. The minimal number of degrees of freedom of the χ^2 statistics is the argument of the parameter ρ function crossing the selected threshold level, marked with dashed black line in Fig. 6.10. To be sure that the condition $\rho > 0.95$ is fulfilled in cases of all positions along the strip, the value equal to 8 is selected for further studies.

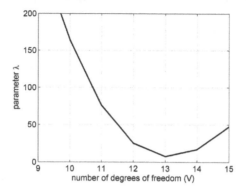

Figure 6.11. Parameter λ calculated for different numbers of degrees of freedom.

The hypothesis of normality was tested for numbers of degrees of freedom ranging from 8 to 15. The comparison of the experimental distribution with the theoretical one was performed based on the statistical test r defined in Eq. (4.24). Figure 6.11 presents results for the data collected by the irradiation of the edge of the scintillator strip. The λ parameter is shown as a function of V degrees of freedom of the theoretical χ^2 and the minimum value of λ is obtained for 13 degrees of freedom. Similar results were obtained for all positions of the irradiation. From this analysis one infers that the 15-dimensional vector in each data set may be approximated with 13 independent and normally distributed variables. We will follow this assumption and investigate a simple hit-position reconstruction method based on a MVN distribution of signals.

Reconstruction is equivalent to the qualification of the 15-dimensional vector to one of the predefined data sets established for the various positions along the scintillator. Figure 6.12 shows an example of the position reconstruction for the 15-dimensional vector created by the γ hitting at center position (black square). The distances d to all data sets are evaluated according to Eq. (4.21), and are marked in Fig. 6.12 as gray circles. The reconstructed position is given as the one for which distance d acquires a minimum (black circle). In this example the reconstruction procedure yielded a hit-position different by 1.8 cm from the true position. It should be noted that the reconstructed position does not have to be limited to the 0.6 cm step that results from the number of acquired data sets. For this purpose, the function of distance d around the minimum may be approximated with parabola based on 3 positions (see

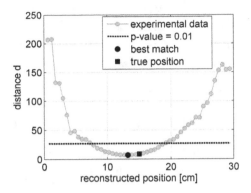

Figure 6.12. Example of position reconstruction for a γ photon interacting in the center of the scintillator.

Fig. 6.12). The reconstructed position may be then calculated as the argument of the minimum of evaluated square function. Knowing that the distance d is derived from χ^2 distribution with 13 degrees of freedom, the p-value of the assignment of the vector to the best-matching data set may be evaluated. The black dotted line in Fig. 6.12 indicates the maximum acceptable distance, equal 27.7, corresponding to the p-value threshold of 0.01. The statistical significance of the assignment of a given measurement to the best-matching data set allows to reject distorted data, e.g., produced by multiple interactions of γ photons in different positions.

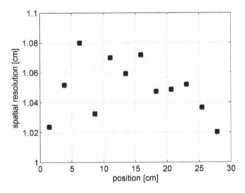

Figure 6.13. The spatial resolution as a function of position along the scintillator strip.

In Fig. 6.13, the resulting spatial resolution, defined as a standard deviation, is presented as a function of irradiated position. From Fig. 6.13, one can infer that the spatial resolution is almost independent of the position of irradiation. An average resolution of the position reconstruction along the strip was determined to be 1.05 cm. In comparison, the proposed method using the lowest threshold (0.06 V) alone, under the same experimental conditions, gives 1.08 cm (standard deviation) spatial resolution.

6.3.2 Hit-position reconstruction using recovered signals

The application of CS theory enables to take an advantage from fully recovered signals and opens an area for new approaches for the reconstruction of position along the strip in the J-PET scanner. However, our preliminary studies reveal that direct application of the recovered waveforms of the signal does not improve the spatial resolution. In fact, due to the low number of photons that reach the photomultipliers, charge, as well as amplitude, of signals is subject to a large variations. In order to improve the spatial resolution, a method of signal normalization that permits to decrease the smearing of signals charge was proposed [3]. The procedure of signal normalization is as follows.

For each training data set of fully sampled signals, mean values of charges at PM1 and PM2 are calculated and saved as $Q_{i(L)}$ and $Q_{i(R)}$, respectively, where $i = 1, ..., L$. Consider a pair of recovered signals $\hat{y}_{(L)}$ and $\hat{y}_{(R)}$ at PM1 and PM2, respectively. The charges of the recovered signals, denoted hereafter as $\hat{Q}_{(L)}$ and $\hat{Q}_{(R)}$, are evaluated as an integrations of the $\hat{y}_{(L)}$ and $\hat{y}_{(R)}$, respectively. The initial classification of the new measurement $\hat{y}_{(L)}$ and $\hat{y}_{(R)}$ to one of the data sets is based on the analysis of distances $d^{(i)}$ (see Eq. (4.21)), as in previous studies in section 6.3. Next, the index j for which the distance d acquires a minimum is selected and the recovered signals are normalized according to the formula:

$$\hat{y}_{n(L)} = \frac{Q_{j(L)}}{\hat{Q}_{(L)}} \hat{y}_{(L)} \tag{6.1}$$

$$\hat{y}_{n(R)} = \frac{Q_{j(R)}}{\hat{Q}_{(R)}} \hat{y}_{(R)}. \tag{6.2}$$

Experimental charge distributions of signals registered via scope are shown in Fig. 6.14. As expected, the mean values are symmetrical with respect to the center of the strip, i.e., position of 15 cm. The estimated average value of charge for center position is 56 pC. The standard deviation along the scintillator strip, not shown in Fig. 6.14, is almost constant and takes the value of about 10 pC.

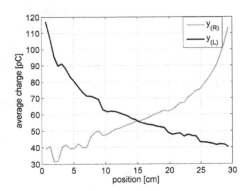

Figure 6.14. Charge distributions along the scintillator strip.

The recovered and normalized signals are further processed in order to extract the hit-position information. Unlike the previous case, when only eight directly registered samples per signal were used, the reconstruction based on fully recovered waveforms required more attention in the establishment of data representation. The concept of concatenation of signals registered in coincidence is illustrated in Fig. 6.15. The signals are al-

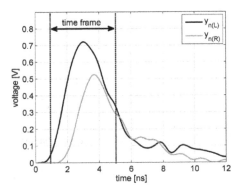

Figure 6.15. Construction of input data for hit-position reconstruction using the recovered pair of signals.

ligned on the timescale taking into account the absolute acquisition time on the voltage levels on both ends of the scintillator strip. The timescale is shifted to the beginning of the signal that arrived first to the photomultiplier (marked in black in Fig. 6.15), since only the relative times are essential. As described in section 6.1.1, for each recovered signal, sample number 20 is used for triggering purposes. In case of the signal that arrived first, the sample at the lowest voltage level corresponds to time 1 ns. This sample indicates the start of the time frame for signal analysis marked with dotted vertical lines in Fig. 6.15. The concatenated, output signal consists of two fragments of recovered signals in selected time frame: first half from $\hat{y}_{n(L)}$ and second half from $\hat{y}_{n(R)}$. In the example shown in Fig. 6.15 the time frame lasts 4 ns and output signal has 160 samples.

The spatial resolutions derived from the recovered signals as a function of the length of the time frames are shown in Fig. 6.16. We have conducted the experiments for time frames of different lengths and for two types of signals: recovered $\hat{y}_{(L)}, \hat{y}_{(R)}$ (marked with a gray curve in Fig. 6.16), recovered and normalized $\hat{y}_{n(L)}, \hat{y}_{n(R)}$ (marked with a black curve in Fig. 6.16). We have carried out the test on the same data set and under the same conditions as described previously in section 6.3, where the average spatial resolution along the strip was about 1.05 cm (black dotted line in Fig. 6.16).

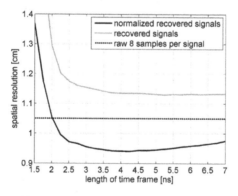

Figure 6.16. Influence of length of the time frame on the spatial resolution using recovered signals.

In Fig. 6.16 it is shown that the application of the recovered signals without normalization does not improve the spatial resolution; the best value is about 1.12 cm. On the other hand, after the signal normalization, the spatial resolution is considerably enhanced. During the optimization procedure, the time frame length was adjusted to 4 ns, which corresponds to the average spatial resolution along the strip of about 0.94 cm (black curve in Fig. 6.16). This result is about 0.1 cm better in comparison to the one evaluated based on signals in the voltage domain alone (black dotted line in Fig. 6.16). It should be stressed that using more than four voltage levels does not lead to significant improvements. The spatial resolution derived from the original signal sampled with a scope is equal to 0.93 cm.

6.4 Prediction of theoretical resolutions of the J-PET scanner

In this part we investigate the accuracy of the method for prediction of the time resolution, i.e., the CRT of the J-PET detector. The model is validated by performing the experiment with a single detection module of the J-PET scanner described in section 6.1.1. In our studies in previous section 6.3, it was shown that the spatial resolution, and thus time resolution, is fairly independent of the irradiation position (see Fig. 6.13 for details). Hence, in the following we determine both experimental and theoretical values of CRTs of the J-PET scanner in one position, at the center of the strip (15 cm). The values of CRT are calculated based on the data set of training signals registered in coincidence at photomultipliers output.

The experimental value of the time resolution is evaluated in a similar way as in the case of previously discussed spatial resolution. In the first step, for each pair of fully sampled signals from the left and right ends of the strip, $\tilde{y}_{(L)}$ and $\tilde{y}_{(R)}$, we simulate a front-end electronic device probing signals at four voltage levels, both at the rising and falling slope. Next, the signals $\hat{y}_{(L)}$ and $\hat{y}_{(R)}$ are recovered using eight samples of signals $\tilde{y}_{(L)}$ and $\tilde{y}_{(R)}$ registered by an oscilloscope, according to the procedure descried in section 4.2. For each pair of the recovered signals $\hat{y}_{(L)}$ and $\hat{y}_{(R)}$, the reconstruction of time $(\hat{\Theta})$ and position $(\hat{z})$ of interaction in the strip is pursued by minimization of the function W in Eq. (4.27). The standard deviation of the empirical distribution of time (σ_Θ), evaluated based on the data set of registered signals, was equal to 80 ps. The corresponding value of CRT, calculated based on Eq. (4.47) was equal to 275 ps. This value of CRT will be treated as the reference for the proposed, theoretical model.

According to the description of the theoretical model in Eq. (4.35), the evaluation of the σ_Θ and time resolution of the PET detector requires determination of the parameter α_2 and covariance matrix S. The values of these parameters vary for different types of applied photomultipliers and are also sensitive to the position of the γ photon interaction along the scintillator strip.

In order to calculate the α_2, the distribution of time of photon registration at the photomultiplier (f_{t_r}) has to be evaluated. In particular the parameters of three pdf functions f_{t_e}, f_{t_p} and f_{t_d}, defined in Eq. (4.2), (4.4) and (4.6), respectively, must be known. It should be stressed that only the last pdf function, f_{t_d}, describes the unique properties of a given type of the photomultiplier. The standard deviation σ_d is delivered by the photomultiplier's producer, for Hamamatsu R4998 photomultiplier $\sigma_d = 68$ ps, and for MCP photomultiplier $\sigma_d = 40$ ps. The values of τ_d, τ_r, σ_e of the f_{t_e} pdf function were adjusted based on the experimental studies with a single BC-420 scintillator strip. The parameter β in Eq. (4.8) was selected in such way that the amplitude of the theoretical signal y is equal to the mean amplitude of signals registered at the center of the strip (15 cm). The analytical solution for f_{t_r} function is difficult to find due to the internal convolution in f_{t_e} function (see Eq. (4.2)). Therefore, the numerical evaluation of a convolution operation was applied. In this work we are interested only in derivation of the CRT of the J-PET detector and we assume that the position of the γ photon interaction is known exactly (see Eq. (4.33)). Therefore, for a fixed position of the interaction at the center of the strip, the signal y may be shifted along the time axis due to the time uncertainty $\Delta\Theta$. In order to evaluate α_2, the parameter $\Delta\Theta$ was changed in the range from -1 to 1 ns. For each value of $\Delta\Theta$, function $W(\Delta\Theta, 0)$ was evaluated based on the shape of theoretical signal y. The resulting function $W(\Delta\Theta, 0)$ is presented in Fig. 6.17[1] with black curve (see also Eq. (4.27)).

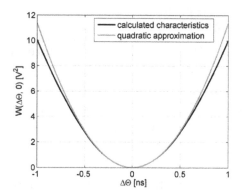

Figure 6.17. The shape of function $W(\Delta\Theta, 0)$ near to the minimum.

According to Eq. (4.33), the function $W(\Delta\Theta, 0)$ may be approximated near $\Delta\Theta = 0$ with the quadratic function. The quadratic approximation

---

of the $W(\Delta\Theta, 0)$ function is marked in Fig. 6.17 with the gray curve and the coefficient of the second order polynomial function is equal to $11.2\ \frac{V^2}{ns^2}$.

The signal y consists of N_p Gaussian shaped signals of single photoelectrons. The number N_p depends on the quantum efficiency of the photomultiplier. In the following we will briefly recall the main results of our earlier works, enabling us to estimate properly the number N_p. The light yield of plastic scintillators amounts to about 10,000 photons per 1 MeV of deposited energy. The 511 keV γ photon may deposit a maximum of 341 keV via Compton scattering [30], which corresponds to the emission of about 3,410 photons. On the other hand, in order to decrease the noise due to scattering of a γ photon inside patient's body, a minimum energy deposition of about 200 keV is required [17]. Therefore, the range of the number of emitted photons discussed hereafter in this chapter is 2,000–3,410. Experiments conducted with Hamamatsu R4998 photomultipliers have revealed that about 280 photoelectrons are produced from the emission of 3,410 photons [17]. According to the preselected range (2,000 to 3,410 photons), the average number of emitted photons is about 2,700. This number corresponds to $N_p = 220$ registered photoelectrons. Since the CRT of the J-PET system will be determined at the center of the strip, the numbers of photoelectrons N_p contributing to the signals induced on the left and right scintillator ends are the same, and are equal to 110.[2]

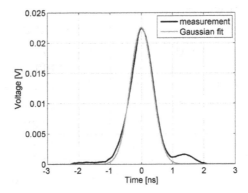

Figure 6.18. An example of the signal of single photoelectron acquired with Hamamatsu R4998 photomultiplier (black curve) and its Gaussian fit (gray curve).

---

[2] L. Raczyński et al., Calculation of the time resolution of the J-PET tomograph using kernel density estimation, *Phys. Med. Biol.* **62** (2017) 5086–5088.

In Fig. 6.18[3] an example of the single photoelectron signal registered with Hamamatsu R4998 photomultiplier and its Gaussian fit are shown. The signals are marked with black and gray curves, respectively. In the acquired signal (black curve) the two Gaussian are observed, however the second one is much smaller and its influence on the calculated parameters is negligible. The standard deviation σ_p of the Gaussian function is about 300 ps and this value is consistent with results presented in report [80].

6.4.1   Noise covariance prediction comparative studies

In this section, a detailed study of the approximation method of components of the covariance matrix S_p, i.e., $\mathrm{Var}(\tilde{y}(n))$ and $\mathrm{Bias}(\tilde{y}(n))$, will be carried out. The proposed method, see Eq. (4.44) and (4.45), will be compared with the well known approximation technique based on the Taylor series expansion, see Eq. (4.42) and (4.43). As the reference for the results of both analytical approaches, the Monte Carlo (MC) simulation will be provided.

In Fig. 6.19, the theoretical signal y at the center of the strip, evaluated from Eq. (4.8), is presented. Additionally, examples of signals $\tilde{y}$, calculated, according to Eq. (4.36), as sum of $N_p = 220$ photoelectrons are shown. In all three cases, we use Gaussian function for model of single photoelectron signals. The three different curves are obtained with standard deviations $\sigma_p = 100, 300, 750$ ps, and are marked with blue, red and green colours, respectively.

The MC simulation was carried out for the constant number of photoelectrons $N_p = 220$, registered by the Hamamatsu R4998 photomultiplier. In order to simulate the $\mathrm{Var}(\tilde{y}(n))$ and $\mathrm{Bias}(\tilde{y}(n))$, only one timestamp of the theoretical signal y, corresponding to the maximum value of 0.6 V (see Fig. 6.19), was used. The analysis of the maximum value in signal y allows one to evaluate the main contribution in the covariance matrix S_p, the location of maximum value of the signal y corresponds to the location of maximum value on diagonal of the covariance matrix S_p. The maximum value of the theoretical signal y is observed in the sample $n = 60$ (see Fig. 6.19). In the first step of MC simulation the random values of photons registration times t_r^k ($k = 1, 2, ..., N_p$) were selected according to the f_{t_r} distribution. Next, the values of all N_p functions $\tilde{y}_k(60)$ were evaluated based on the Eq. (4.37) and summed up giving $\tilde{y}(60)$. The examples of samples $\tilde{y}(60)$ calculated for three different standard deviations

---

[3] © Institute of Physics and Engineering in Medicine. Reproduced by permission of IOP Publishing. All rights reserved.

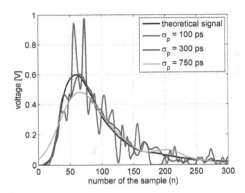

Figure 6.19. Signals observed on the photomultiplier output generated by interaction in the center of the scintillator strip; theoretical signal y (see Eq. (4.8)) is marked with the black curve, examples of signals $\tilde{y}$ (see Eq. (4.36)) simulated for $N_p = 220$ photoelectrons and three different standard deviation $\sigma_p = 100, 300, 750$ ps, are marked with blue, red, and green colours, respectively.

$\sigma_p = 100, 300, 750$ ps, are marked with full blue, red, and green squares in Fig. 6.19, respectively. The abovementioned procedure was repeated 10^6 times for different values of σ_p from 50 ps to 750 ps with step of 25 ps. The range of σ_p has been selected after preliminary calculations taking into account the expected number of registered photoelectrons in the J-PET scenario.

The reference values of $\mathrm{Bias}^2(\tilde{y}(60))$ and $\mathrm{Var}(\tilde{y}(60))$, obtained with MC simulation, are marked with black dotted curves in Fig. 6.20.[4] An approximation of $\mathrm{Var}(\tilde{y})$ for the proposed method and method based on the Taylor series expansion (black and gray curves, respectively) are very similar to the reference curve for small values and tend to differ for larger values of σ_p. However, in the most interesting region, for σ_p equal to about 300 ps, the proposed method is more accurate than the Taylor series based method and the values of $\mathrm{Var}(\tilde{y})$ are equal to 6.5×10^{-3} V^2 and 7.0×10^{-3} V^2, respectively (the reference value of $\mathrm{Var}(\tilde{y})$ from MC simulation is equal to 5.1×10^{-3} V^2). Comparison of the $\mathrm{Bias}^2(\tilde{y})$ and $\mathrm{Var}(\tilde{y})$ curves reveals the fundamental relation between variance and bias. The variance dominates for smaller values of σ_p and becomes comparable with bias for σ_p at the level of about 450 ps (compare two reference dotted curves in Fig. 6.20a and 6.20b). For σ_p larger than 450 ps, the total error is mostly influenced by the bias. It is worth noting that in that case the Taylor series based method significantly underestimates the values of

---

[4]

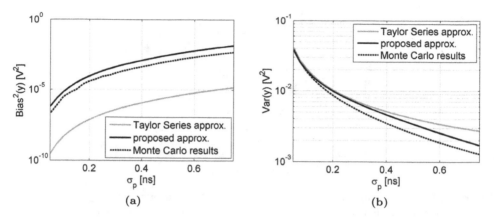

Figure 6.20. The comparison of estimation of $\mathrm{Bias}^2[\tilde{y}]$ (a) and $\mathrm{Var}[\tilde{y}]$ (b) with two analytical approaches: the proposed one (black curve), and the one based on the Taylor series expansion (gray curve). The reference characteristics was obtained with the MC simulation (black dotted curve).

$\mathrm{Bias}^2(\tilde{y})$, see Fig. 6.20a, which leads to the underestimation of the overall error.[5]

6.4.2   Calculation of theoretical CRTs of different J-PET systems

In the following we analyze the value of time resolution as a function of the number of registered photoelectrons (N_p) and standard deviation of the single photoelectron signal (σ_p). As discussed in the previous section, for each number N_p it is possible to find the optimal value of σ_p, for which the smallest sum of $\mathrm{Bias}^2(\tilde{y})$ and $\mathrm{Var}(\tilde{y})$ is observed. For instance, for $N_p = 220$, the optimal σ_p, denoted hereafter as $\sigma_{p(opt)}$, is about 430 ps (see Fig. 6.21). In the case of Hamamatsu R4998 photomultiplier, the σ_p is not a variable and has fixed value of about 300 ps. However, the MCP photomultiplier registers timestamps of the signal instead of the complete signal. Therefore, the value of $\sigma_{p(opt)}$ of each contributing signal may be adjusted accordingly to the number of registered timestamps (N_p). In that sense, the optimization of the $\sigma_{p(opt)}$ value for MCP photomultiplier may be provided. In general, the MCP photomultiplier is capable of registering all the timestamps of the photons reaching the scintillator end. In order to account for possible inefficiency of the MCP, we determine the characteristics of the J-PET equipped with the MCP in the range

---

[5] L. Raczyński et al., Calculation of the time resolution of the J-PET tomograph using kernel density estimation, *Phys. Med. Biol.* **62** (2017) 5089–5090.

$100 \leqslant N_p \leqslant 700$. The highest number, $N_p = 700$ indicates the maximum number of registered photoelectrons in the experimental scenario, and was selected in order to demonstrate the best theoretical resolution of J-PET. The characteristics describing the optimal standard deviation ($\sigma_{p(opt)}$) for different N_p is shown in Fig. 6.21. As expected, the larger the number of registered photoelectrons the smaller the value of $\sigma_{p(opt)}$. The theory of kernel density estimation [81, 105] implies that as the N_p goes to infinity, the $\sigma_{p(opt)}$ approaches zero.

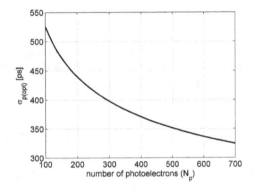

Figure 6.21. Optimal standard deviation ($\sigma_{p(opt)}$) of single photoelectron signal as a function of number of registered photoelectrons.

The procedure for calculation of the theoretical CRT for MCP photomultiplier is as follows. First, for a given number N_p, the optimal value of $\sigma_{p(opt)}$ was estimated based on the characteristics shown in Fig. 6.21. In case of MCP photomultiplier, the output signal is given directly, based on the measured timestamps and assumed model of the single photoelectron signal. Therefore, the recovery procedure is not needed and covariance matrix $S = S_p$ (see Eq. (4.13) for details); the matrix S_p is calculated based on the proposed model, described in Eqs (4.44) and (4.45). Next, σ_Θ is evaluated based on Eq. (4.35) and finally the CRT is calculated according to Eq. (4.47).

The resulting characteristic of CRT is depicted with black solid curve in Fig. 6.22.[6] The presented values of CRT take into account an additional smearing of the time due to the unknown depth of interaction in a scintillator strip with a thickness of 19 mm, see Eq. (4.47) for details. The presented results show that the best theoretical CRT of the J-PET scanner with 30 cm long strips is estimated for the MCP photomultiplier

---

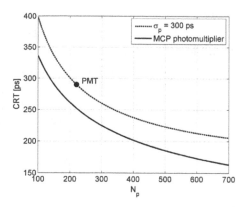

Figure 6.22. Theoretical calculations of the CRT as a function of the number of photo-electrons N_p, of the J-PET detector equipped with MCP and Hamamatsu R4998 photomultipliers.

capable of registering all timestamps of arrival for 700 photons, is at the level of 170 ps. Additionally, the theoretical value of CRT calculated for Hamamatsu R4998 photomultiplier for $N_p = 220$ and $\sigma_p = 300$ ps, also including the S_r matrix describing the signal recovery uncertainity, is marked with full black circle in Fig. 6.22. Our calculation shows that the application of the proposed prediction method can give a very similar result to the experimental value; instead of 275 ps, the theoretical model gave CRT $= 290$ ps. The obtained results demonstrate that the quantum efficiency (equivalent to the number N_p), is one of the most important factors influencing the overall performance of the PET scanner.[7]

As shown in [19], the second factor influencing the time resolution is the photomultipliers transit time spread. According to the results shown in Fig. 6.23, there is a negligible dependence of the CRT on the transit time spread value. For fixed value of the parameter describing the quantum efficiency of Hamamatsu R4998 photomultiplier, that corresponds to registration of $N_p = 220$ photoelectrons on average, in the selected range from 20 ps to 160 ps of photomultiplier's transit time spread, the CRT of the J-PET detector differs by 5 ps (see Fig. 6.23 for details).

---

[7] L. Raczyński et al., Calculation of the time resolution of the J-PET tomograph using kernel density estimation, *Phys. Med. Biol.* **62** (2017) 5090−5092.

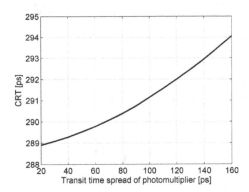

Figure 6.23. Theoretical calculations of the CRT as a function of photomultiplier transit time spread.

6.5   Event classification in the J-PET detector

This section starts the presentation of results of high-level data processing in the J-PET scanner. From this moment, all the information concerning the signals acquired at the photomultipliers output is encapsuled in the form of events. As mentioned in section 5.1, each event is described with six features and is treated as a point in 6-D space. In this section we will visualize and provide a simple analysis of the distribution of all three types of events, i.e., true, scattered and random, by using SOM. We will focus on the data from MC simulation described in section 6.1.3, since only in this case exact information about different event types is available.

Before the application of the SOM, the input data set of events was reduced. The goal of this preselection step was the rejection of the events from outside of the detector field of view. For this purpose two selection criteria were applied. First, the field of view of the J-PET scanner in transverse direction, i.e., (x, y) cross-section, was limited to the circle with diameter equal to 60 cm. Secondly, reconstructed position of event along the axial direction, i.e., z coordinate, was limited to $\pm$ 20 cm. Consequently, total number of 50.0 million coincident events was reduced to 33.3 million. This number included 20.0 million trues (100% of initial number), 9.3 million scatters (99% of initial number) and 4.0 million randoms (20% of initial number). It should be stressed that only the number of random events changed significantly after the preselection step.

6.5.1   Dimensionality reduction using SOM

The first investigation concerns the analysis of quality of the dimensionality reduction using SOM network. This study is conducted according to the description given in section 5.1.2. The data set containing 33.3 million events is divided into two disjoint subsets: training and testing parts, with a ratio 4:1, respectively. The 6-D training data set is subjected to the input of the SOM network. The Gaussian neighbourhood function, with initial standard deviation equal 2, is applied (see Eq. (3.17) for details). During the learning process, the standard deviation shrinks with time, to achieve finally the value of 0.4 after 1000 epochs. We conduct trainings of the SOM maps with different number of neurons (N_g^2) in the square grid, with N_g in range from 16 to 112 in steps of 16. For each trained network with N_g^2 neurons, a quantization error (q_e) is evaluated. An empirical dependence of the $\log_2(q_e)$ on the $\log_2(N_g)$ is marked with a dark gray curve in Fig. 6.24 and may be accurately approximated with linear function according to Eq. (5.3).

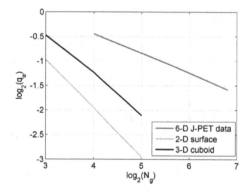

Figure 6.24. Dependence of the quantization error (q_e) on the size of the neural network map (N_g) for three data sets in loglog scale.

The parameter κ defined in Eq. (5.3), describing the slope factor of the dark gray line, is about 0.41. In order to provide the parameter κ for data sets that can be visualized, we perform additionally the experiments with two synthetic data sets presented in Fig. 6.25. In both cases, the 3-D input synthetic data are marked with small, gray circles and positions of the neurons in the trained SOM are marked with black circles.

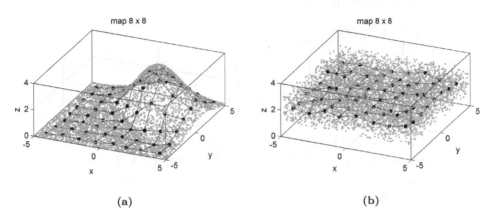

Figure 6.25. Example of visualization of 2-D non-linear surface (a) and 3-D cuboid (b) by 2-D SOM.

The data set in Fig. 6.25a describes the non-linear surface $z(x, y)$

$$z(x, y) = \max(2(x + y) \cdot \exp\left((-x^2 - y^2)/10\right), 0) \qquad (6.3)$$

while the data set in Fig. 6.25b is a cuboid of size $10 \times 10 \times 2$ (the units in both cases are arbitrary). During the learning process the Gaussian neighbourhood function with the same parameters as for J-PET data was applied. In both instances the number of neurons in the grid in each direction was changed from 8 to 32 (see Fig. 6.24). The dependencies of the $\log_2(q_e)$ on the $\log_2(N_g)$ for synthetic data sets from Figs 6.25a and 6.25b are marked with a light gray and black curves in Fig. 6.24, respectively. In case of non-linear surface $z(x, y)$, the parameter κ evaluated based on linear fit of the empirical values in Fig. 6.24 is about 0.99. The value of κ almost equal 1 corresponds to very accuarate fit of the SOM grid on 3-D space occupied by the data set (see Fig. 6.25a for details). On the other hand, the κ calculated for the cuboid data set is about 0.82. However, still quite reasonable presentation of the input 3-D data on the 2-D SOM grid is obtained. It is clear that the quality of this fit is highly associated with the thickness of the cuboid (which in our example is 2). The greater the thickness of the cuboid, the smaller the value of κ. Since the parameter κ describing the coplanarity of the 6-D J-PET data is about 0.41, the results presented in the next section are only indicative.

6.5.2   Event classification using SOM

As mentioned, coincidence events are classified into three types: true, scattered and random. While the true events are desirable, the scattered and random coincidences contribute to the background and hinder the reconstruction process, degrading image quality. In the following, we consider true events as positive cases (P), and both scattered and random events as negative (N) cases. In order to measure the quality of classification, we calculate two parameters: true positive rate (TPR) and positive predictive value (PPV). The TPR and PPV measure sensitivity and precision of the classification, respectively, and are defined as in statistical classification, i.e.,

$$\text{TPR} = \frac{\text{TP}}{\text{TP} + \text{FN}} \tag{6.4}$$

$$\text{PPV} = \frac{\text{TP}}{\text{TP} + \text{FP}}. \tag{6.5}$$

The goal of the event selection is to maximize the classification precision (PPV) for assumed sensitivity (TPR) close to 1. In futher analysis, we agree to discard 5% of total number of true events (TPR = 95%) and we investigate the value of PPV parameter for different classifiers.

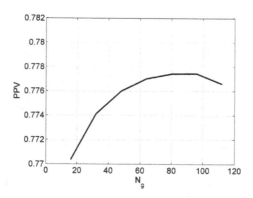

Figure 6.26. Influence of the size of the SOM map grid (N_g) on the classification precision (PPV). The parameter PPV is evaluated for fixed value of TPR = 95%.

In Fig. 6.26 the influence of the size of the SOM on the precision of event classification is presented. As described in the previous section, we conduct trainings of different SOMs with square grid, where N_g was changed in range from 16 to 112 in steps of 16. The results shown in Fig. 6.26 indicate that the optimal classification conditions occur for $N_g = 96$, where the PPV reaches the maximal value of about 0.777.

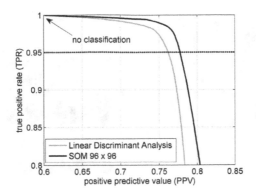

Figure 6.27. Comparison of performance of SOM classifier and Linear Discriminant Analysis.

In Fig. 6.27 the performance of the best SOM classifier with 96×96 neurons and the reference Linear Discriminant Analysis (LDA) method [106] is compared. It should be stressed that if no classification is provided, all true events are considered (TPR $= 1$), while the initial precision (PPV) is about 0.60, since the total number of 33.3 million coincident events includes 20.0 million trues. This point is common for curves describing both methods, and is marked with an arrow in Fig. 6.27. The analysis of the characteristics of TPRs as functions of PPVs shows that the SOM classifier achieves slightly better results than the reference LDA algorithm in wide range of parameter variability. For selected threshold of TPR $= 95\%$, indicated with black dotted line in Fig. 6.27, the PPV is about 0.762 and 0.777 for LDA and SOM, respectively.

As mentioned, the SOM enables visualization of high-dimensional feature space, 6-D in case of J-PET events, by creating low-dimensional 2-D views. Fig. 6.28 illustrates the pdfs in form of images in all three event classes. The images have the size of the optimal SOM map, i.e., 96×96 neurons. Higher values of intensity in images in Fig. 6.28 indicate the areas of concentration of each class. For instance, it may be seen that true and random events are located in different parts of the map and it is much easier to distinguish between true and random events than true and scattered events.

As described in section 5.1.3, the SOM map allows the events classification based on maximal conditional probability. Hence, in each position on the map (i, j), the class with maximal $\mathbb{P}(c_k|W_{ij})$ (see Eq. (5.4)) may be indicated. The division of the 2-D SOM map based on maximal probability $\mathbb{P}(c_k|W_{ij})$ for three event classes is shown in Fig. 6.29 (left). The

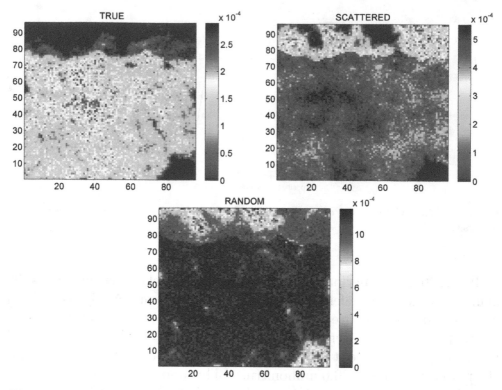

Figure 6.28. Visualization of pdfs of 3 event classes on 2-D SOM with 96 × 96 neurons.

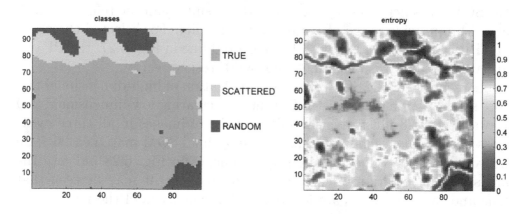

Figure 6.29. Division of three event classes (left) and corresponding information entropy (right) on SOM map with 96 × 96 neurons.

largest area in the center of the map is covered by the true events (blue colour). Moreover, a specific two colour mosaic of green and red colours (scattered and random events) is observed at the top of the map. However, taking into account the information entropy from Fig. 6.29 (right), the best classification conditions occur for random events marked with red colour in Fig. 6.29 (left). In this case, most of pixels in corresponding area in the entropy map in Fig. 6.29 (right) have values close to 0. On the other hand, the entropy takes maximal value for pixel (i, j), where the conditional probability $\mathbb{P}(c_k|W_{ij}) = 1/3$ for each class is 1.099. The highest values of entropy are observed on the borders between different event types.

6.6 Image reconstruction using Total Variation regularization

In this section the last part of high-level data processing in the J-PET scanner, namely the image reconstruction, will be discussed. The reconstruction method, introduced in section 5.2, is validated using the standards for medical diagnostic imaging equipment published by the NEMA, the association of electrical equipment and medical imaging manufacturers in the United States. In the view of presented studies, the most important NEMA standard is NEMA-NU-2-2012 [101], which pertains to PET devices. This norm comprehensively defines the characteristics of PET scanners, e.g., the spatial resolution, the image quality. The NEMA characteristics will be delivered to both experimental and MC simulation data. In the first step, in section 6.6.1, we provide a detailed study of the performance and optimization of the proposed image reconstruction algorithm using simulation data from the NEMA IEC body phantom. Next, in sections 6.6.2 and 6.6.3 we investigate the reconstruction of the experimental data acquired with the prototype 3-layer J-PET detector. In particular, in section 6.6.2, we demonstrate that the proposed imaging technique allows the estimation of the CRT of the prototype J-PET system.

6.6.1 Reconstruction of NEMA IEC body phantom

Processing using simulation data allows flexibility in selection of the event types considered in image reconstruction. As mentioned in section 6.1.3, a total number of registered events for the NEMA IEC simulation study equals 50.0 million coincident events and includes 20.0 million trues. During the investigation shown in this section, only true coincidence events are considered in the reconstruction process and the other two types of events, namely scattered and random, are excluded from the event list. Therefore, only multiplicative factors, i.e., attenuation and detector geometric sensitivity, are considered at the pre-correction step. The attenuation correction is performed using the attenuation map used for the GATE simulation.

Reconstructions of simulated data are performed in MATLAB 7.14.0 (R2012a) with the use of chosen procedures from the Image Processing Toolbox. The proposed reconstruction algorithm based on TV minimization was implemented based on the work of [61], details of this approach are presented in section 3.2.1. The reconstructed images are represented as 3-D matrices with the voxel size of $0.25 \times 0.25 \times 0.25$ cm^3.

The performance of the reconstruction was evaluated using two image quality assessments defined in the NEMA-NU-2-2012 standard: contrast recovery coefficient (CRC) and background variability (BV). In the transaxial slice through the centers of hot and cold spheres, a circular region of interest (ROI) was defined on each sphere. Twelve circular ROIs of appropriate diameter were then defined on the phantom background. These background ROIs were automatically replicated to four transaxial slices ±10 mm and ±20 mm on either side of the central slice. Thus, in total, 60 ROIs were defined on the phantom background for each sphere. The CRC for each hot sphere with diameter d was calculated as:

$$\mathrm{CRC}_H = \frac{C_{H,d}/C_{B,d} - 1}{4 - 1}, \qquad (6.6)$$

where $C_{H,d}$ was the average count in the hot sphere, $C_{B,d}$ was the average of the background ROI counts and 4 was the true activity ratio between the hot spheres and the warm background. The CRC for each cold sphere with diameter d was calculated as:

$$\mathrm{CRC}_C = 1 - C_{C,d}/C_{B,d}, \qquad (6.7)$$

where $C_{C,d}$ was the average count in the cold sphere. The BV for each sphere with diameter d was calculated as:

$$\mathrm{BV} = \frac{S_d}{C_{B,d}}, \qquad (6.8)$$

where S_d was the standard deviation of the background ROI counts. Additionally, a root mean square error (RMSE) between the full 3-D reconstructed image ($\hat{\mathbf{f}}$) and the true phantom activity image ($\mathbf{f}^0$) was calculated as a global quality criterion taking into account both bias and variance of the reconstruction algorithms:

$$\text{RMSE} = \sqrt{\frac{1}{N}\sum_{i=1}^{N}\left(\hat{\mathbf{f}}_i - \mathbf{f}_i^0\right)^2}. \qquad (6.9)$$

Shift-invariance violation investigation

In the first step of the analysis the influence of the θ_{acc} angle value on the performance of the proposed algorithm was investigated. For assumed size of cylindrical J-PET detector $\theta_{\text{max}} \approx 30.3^o$. Additionally, taking into account the axial (90 mm) and transaxial (150 mm) extent of the NEMA IEC body phantom, θ_{min} that satisfies shift-invariance equals 15.5^o [96]. θ_{acc} was changed in the range from 15° to 30° with 2.5^o step. Table 6.1 lists in the second column the percentage of total counts as a function of θ_{acc} for a total of 20.0 million true events.

Table 6.1. Performance of the proposed method for different values of θ_{acc} angle.

θ_{acc} [^{o}]	% of total	min(RMSE)
15.0	63.1	0.028
17.5	74.2	0.026
20.0	83.4	0.025
22.5	90.6	0.024
25.0	95.7	0.026
27.5	98.8	0.028
30.0	100.0	0.030

Figure 6.30 compares the trends in CRC and BV of the 13-mm hot sphere (Fig. 6.30a) and the 22-mm hot sphere (Fig. 6.30b) for three different θ_{acc} values: smallest one (light gray curves), highest one (dark gray curves) and middle one (black curves). The error bars indicate standard deviations and are estimated from the five realizations of event smearing with assumed J-PET resolutions. The resulting curves for the remaining four cases (see Tab. 6.1) were not shown in Fig. 6.30 for the clarity of presentation. Each particular CRC versus BV curve was obtained after applying different regularization parameter μ (see Eq. 5.28). More details about the influence of the parameter μ on the reconstructed image will be discussed in the next section.

For a quantitative comparison of the results for different θ_{acc} angles, for each CRC versus BV curve a minimal RMSE between reconstructed and true image of activity is calculated. The resulting values of min(RMSE)

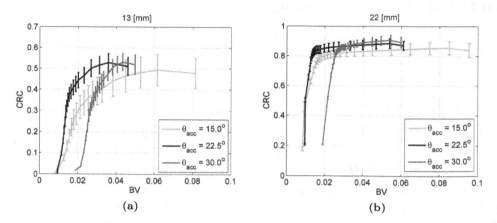

Figure 6.30. CRC versus BV in the reconstructed images of 13 mm hot sphere (a) and 22 mm hot sphere (b) computed for different θ_{acc} values.

are listed in Tab. 6.1 in third column. We observe that the best results are obtained for the $\theta_{\mathrm{acc}} = 22.5^{o}$ (see black curves in Fig. 6.30 and fourth row of Tab. 6.1). Hence, during the comparative studies presented in the next section, we applied $\theta_{\mathrm{acc}} = 22.5^{o}$. This requirement imposes that the proposed TOF-BPTV algorithm uses 90.6% of acquired data (fourth row of Tab. 6.1) that corresponds to about 18.1 million true events.

PET reconstruction comparative studies

To perform the comparative studies of the proposed TOF-BPTV method, the TOF-MLEM algorithm, implemented in CASToR software [107], was applied. CASToR offers several reconstruction algorithms for LM data as well as several data correction techniques such as attenuation correction, normalization and point spread function (PSF) modeling. An iterative TOF-MLEM optimization algorithm using 60 iterations with no subsets division was selected. The TOF-MLEM cost function in CASToR software does not include any prior distribution and therefore the algorithm converges to the noisy image. A few approaches can be applied to remedy this problem and improve the quality of reconstructed images. First possibility is to stop the reconstruction method after given number of iterations and use current image estimate as a solution. Moreover, CASToR applies PSF filters. Our preliminary investigations showed that spatial resolution of the J-PET scanner can be approximated with 3-D Gaussian of 6 mm transaxial FWHM and 12 mm axial FWHM and this kernel was applied to model a shift-invariant PSF in CASToR.

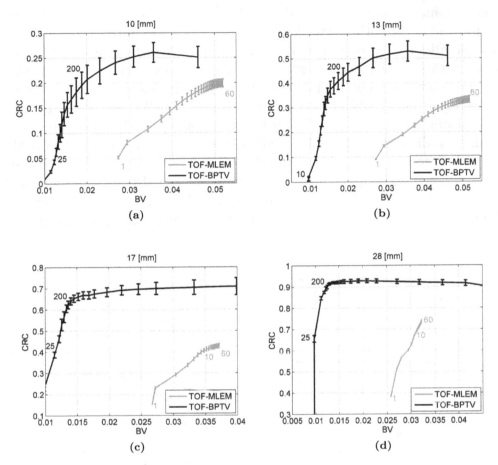

Figure 6.31. CRC versus BV in the reconstructed images of 10 mm hot sphere (a), 13 mm hot sphere (b), 17 mm hot sphere (c) and 28 mm cold sphere (d) computed for TOF-BPTV algorithm (black curves) and TOF-MLEM algorithm (gray curves). Values of μ and iteration number are indicated with black and gray colours, respectively.

Figure 6.31 compares the averages CRC and BV of the hot and cold spheres for both TOF-MLEM and TOF-BPTV image reconstruction. The error bars indicate standard deviations and are estimated from the five realizations of event smearing with assumed J-PET resolutions. In case of TOF-BPTV method the curves were obtained after applying various regularization parameter μ values in a range from 10 to 5000. In case of the TOF-MLEM algorithm the curves were obtained after applying different iterations in the range from 1 to 60. In all cases shown in Fig. 6.31, we observe the typical trade-off between the contrast (CRC) and the noise (BV). The regularization parameter μ trades-off the TV norm and the fidelity term (see Eq. 5.28). Small values of regularization parameter favor TV penalty and give less noisy images, but the result may be smoothed with large bias. In that case both CRC and BV have small values (see Fig. 6.31 for $\mu = 10$ or 25). Increasing value of μ tends to give sharper images, but noise is also amplified (both CRC and BV increase). For each sphere the optimal μ was determined where the CRC reached 95% of its maximum value. In all cases μ was in the range from 200 to 300, and finally the smallest $\mu = 200$ was selected for further studies with TOF-BPTV algorithm. Similarly, for TOF-MLEM algorithm, for each sphere the iteration number was extracted where the CRC reached 95% of its maximum value. For 10-, 13-, 17- and 28-mm spheres the 16th, 15th, 11th and 14th iterations were indicated, respectively. Finally, the 15th iteration was selected for further presentations.

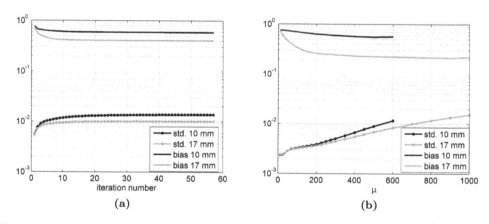

Figure 6.32. Biases and standard deviations of the hot sources with 10 mm and 17 mm diameter for TOF-MLEM algorithm (a) and TOF-BPTV algorithm (b).

Figure 6.32 illustrates bias in the region of the two hot spheres of 10 and 17 mm diameter and the background standard deviation values. The bias is defined as the difference between the true and reconstructed mean value in the ROIs. We normalized the image of true phantom activity to the range from 0 to 1, where 0 means no radioactivity, 1 corresponds to the hot regions and value 0.25 corresponds to the warm background (true activity ratio between the hot spheres and the background is 4). Each reconstructed image was normalized off-line to have the same total sum as the true phantom activity image. It is worth to note that the background standard deviations are approximately the same with TOF-BPTV for selected $\mu = 200$ (see Fig. 6.32b), while differ with TOF-MLEM for the 15th iteration (see Fig. 6.32a). The bias of the smallest source is almost the same for both algorithms, while the bias of the 17 mm diameter sphere is smaller in case of TOF-BPTV algorithm.

In Fig. 6.33 the two exemplary images in the transaxial (top) and coronal (bottom) slices through the centers of all spheres for 15th iteration for TOF-MLEM algorithm (left) and $\mu = 200$ for TOF-BPTV approach (right), are shown. The RMSE between the reconstructed image and the true phantom activity image is equal to 0.024 for TOF-BPTV method and 0.032 for TOF-MLEM algorithm. It can be seen that the structure of the warm phantom background differs and TOF-BPTV image (right) exhibits less intensity variability than the TOF-MLEM image (left). In both images the smallest hot sphere can be distinguished from the warm phantom background.

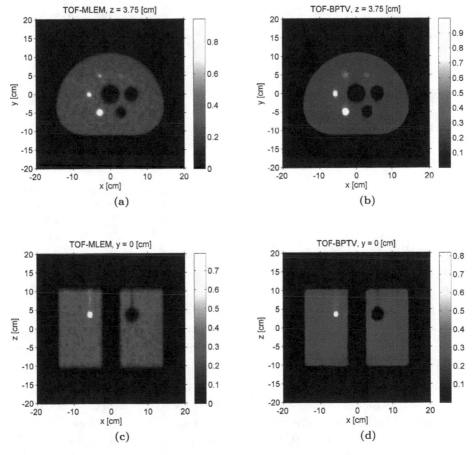

Figure 6.33. Transaxial (top) and coronal (bottom) slices through the centers of spheres inside the NEMA IEC body phantom. Images shown for 15th iteration of TOF-MLEM algorithm (a, c) and reconstructed using TOF-BPTV algorithm with $\mu = 200$ (b, d).

The reduced intensity variability of the TOF-BPTV image can also be clearly seen in the profiles through the images in transaxial slices shown in Fig. 6.34. In case of TOF-MLEM both cold spheres, observed on 90° and 150° in circular profile, have not reached value 0. The circular profiles further indicate that intensities in the TOF-BPTV image in hot spheres are more flat in comparison to the TOF-MLEM image. Therefore, despite the fact that maximal values for two smallest hot spheres, observed on 30° and 330° in circular profile, are higher for TOF-MLEM images, the mean values and CRCs are slightly better for TOF-BPTV algorithm.

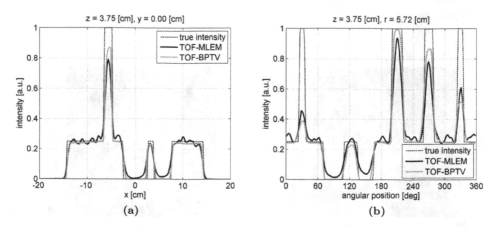

Figure 6.34. Emission density profiles through the reconstructed images in transaxial slices of Fig. 6.33: line profile for $y = 0$ cm (a), circular profile over centers of all spheres for $r = 5.72$ cm (b).

The studies presented in this section do not cover the comparison of computational speed of the TOF-BPTV and TOF-MLEM methods. Since both algorithms are created with different programming languages, namely C++ in case of TOF-MLEM (CASToR) and MATLAB in case of TOF-BPTV, the estimate of efficiency could be only indicative. Additionally, most of the PET reconstruction software does not support multilayer geometry and therefore cannot be applied directly to the experimental data acquired with the 3-layer prototype J-PET detector presented in the next sections. Therefore, in order to perform the comparative studies, including computational speed, of the proposed method, we implemented the TOF-FBP algorithm in MATLAB environment. We start the investigation of the proposed image reconstruction using experimental data acquired with the 3-layer J-PET detector, with estimation of the time resolution of the prototype system.

6.6.2 Estimation of CRT of the prototype J-PET scanner

According to the description of the reconstruction algorithm in section 5.2, the processing starts with deposition of the acquired set of events into the TOF back-projected image. Given an experimental data with point-like source placed in the center of the tomograph, the convolution operator a may be derived directly based on TOF back-projected image (see Eq. (5.18) for details). On the other hand, the operator a holds the information about the CRT (operator $a_{(1)}$ see Eq. (5.23)) and the axial spatial resolution (operator $a_{(3)}$ see Eq. (5.25)). Therefore, given an experimentally derived operator a, it is possible to estimate the time and axial spatial resolutions.

It should be stressed that the time and axial spatial resolutions are related via linear equation [17]:

$$\sigma_z = v_{\mathrm{sc}} \cdot \sigma_\Theta \tag{6.10}$$

where σ_z is standard deviation of Gaussian function describing uncertainty of the measurement along axial position, σ_Θ is standard deviation of Gaussian function describing uncertainty of the measurement of interaction moment, and v_{sc} denotes the effective velocity of the light signal inside the scintillator. Combining Eq. (6.10) with the formula for determining the CRT in Eq. (4.47), we obtain finally:

$$\sigma_z = (2.35\sqrt{2})^{-1} v_{\mathrm{sc}} \sqrt{\mathrm{CRT}^2 - \frac{D^2}{c^2}}. \tag{6.11}$$

The procedure of estimation of the CRT of the prototype J-PET scanner with 192 scintillator strips was as follows. In the first step, the overall data set with 70 million coincident events was TOF back-projected into the image space. In order to compare the empirical operator a with theoretical model described in Eq. (5.22) only one out of six point-like sources, located the nearest to the tomograph center, i.e., in position $(0, 1, 0)$, was retrieved from the data set. For this purpose, the field of view of the J-PET scanner in all three directions was limited to 10 cm and centered at position $(0, 1, 0)$. The resulting image was a 3-D matrice with the voxel size of $0.4 \times 0.4 \times 0.4$ cm^3 and was built of $25 \times 25 \times 25$ voxels. The overall number of events in the resulting cube was about 0.5 million.

We carried out the experiments for different theoretical models of operator a with values of the CRT (operator $a_{(1)}$) from 300 to 700 ps with 20 ps steps. In each case, the standard deviation σ_z in operator $a_{(3)}$ was adjusted according to Eq. (6.11). The overall operator a was calculated as the 3-D image with the same size as the just mentioned empirical TOF back-projected image. In Fig. 6.35, cross-correlation coefficient between

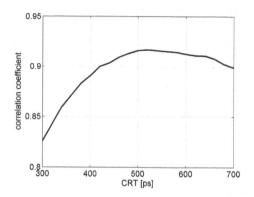

Figure 6.35.   Correlation coefficient between the experimental back-projected image of point source and operators a evaluated for different values of CRT.

empirical and theoretical operators a is plotted as the function of the selected CRT. Cross-correlation coefficient is a similarity measure between two images and its values are in the range from -1 to 1, where 1 corresponds to fully correlated images. From Fig. 6.35 it may be seen that highest cross-correlation value is achieved for the CRT = 520 ps and is about 0.92. It should be stressed that the function is not symmetrical with respect to the estimated value of correct CRT. For smaller CRT the cross-correlation values drop down faster, while for higher CRT the function is more flat. The theoretical CRT of the prototype J-PET scanner derived from this analysis agrees with the experimental CRT value, reported to be about 500 ps [20]. The corresponding standard deviation σ_z of the uncertainty of the measurement of position along the scintillator strip is found based on Eq. (6.11) and is 1.96 cm, where the thickness (D) of the plastic scintillator is 1.9 cm and the speed of light signals in the scintillator (v_{sc}) is 12.6 cm ns^{-1} [17].

6.6.3   Reconstruction of six point-like sources

With the estimated values of the CRT and σ_z of the operator a describing the prototype J-PET detector in hand, the reconstruction of the 3-D image of six point-like sources is provided. Before the reconstruction process, similarly as in the previous study with experimental data, described in section 6.6.2, the total number of 70 million coincident events was TOF back-projected into the image space. The reconstruction volume was limited to the cube centered at position $(0, 0, 0)$ with the size of $50 \times 50 \times 50$ cm^3, and comprising $125 \times 125 \times 125$ voxels. The number of coincident events in the imaging area was 11.2 million. Hence, after limiting the field of view, 58.8 million events were classified as random coincidences and were excluded from further analysis. Since the point-like sources were attached to the styrofoam panel, which has low density, the probability for scattering and attenuation on the panel was negligible. Therefore, only detector geometric sensitivity of the 3-layer J-PET scanner was taken into account for the correction of the reconstructed images.

The performance of the reconstruction of point-like sources was evaluated using the spatial resolution parameter described in the NEMA-NU-2-2012 standard. The spatial resolution of a PET system represents its ability to distinguish between two points after image reconstruction. This parameter characterizes the widths of the reconstructed PSF image of point-like sources. The spatial resolution of the 3-layer prototype J-PET scanner is determined by estimation of the FWHM in the transverse and axial directions of PSF images at six positions inside the detector volume. At each position of the reconstructed image, a voxel with the maximum intensity is found and the 1-D profiles along transverse and axial directions are determined.

PET reconstruction comparative studies

As a reference reconstruction method, TOF-FBP was employed. The TOF-FBP method was implemented in MATLAB according to the description given in [108]. Since the choice of the apodizing function is not unique [109], during our preliminary studies we tested different filters. We observed that the best results are obtained for the Hamming window:

$$W(v_s) = \begin{cases} |v_s| \left(1 + \cos(\pi v_s/v_c)\right)/2 & |v_s| \leq v_c \\ 0 & \text{otherwise} \end{cases} \qquad (6.12)$$

where v_s is the frequency space coordinate associated with s variable (see Eq. 5.8), and v_c is the cut-off frequency which plays the role of regularization parameter. Note that since $W(v_s) \neq 1$, reconstruction yields a biased estimate. It should be stressed that in case of the TOF-FBP method, a trade-off between variance and bias in reconstructed images is optimized by changing the v_c parameter.

The two image reconstruction examples, based on the TOF-FBP algorithm with regularization via apodizing functions and the proposed

TOF-BPTV method, are shown in Fig. 6.36 on the left and right panels, respectively. The TOF-FBP image was obtained for optimal regulariza-

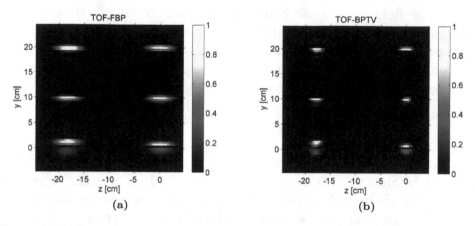

Figure 6.36. Sagittal slices through the centers of six point-like sources ($x = 0$ cm). Images shown for $v_c = 1$ of TOF-FBP algorithm (a), and reconstructed using TOF-BPTV algorithm with $\mu = 200$ (b).

tion parameter $v_c = 1$, i.e., the parameter that minimizes the spatial resolution. In case of the TOF-BPTV algorithm, regularization parameter $\mu = 200$ was selected according to the optimization studies presented in section 6.6.1. It can be seen that the widths of the reconstructed images differ and TOF-BPTV image (right) exhibits better spatial resolution along axial (z) direction than the TOF-FBP image (left). On the other hand, in both images the spatial resolution along y direction is similar. For clarity of presentation the activities of six point-like sources in Fig. 6.36 are normalized to 1.

The estimated PSF values for 3-D reconstruction of point-sources located in six positions for both methods: TOF-FBP (gray solid and dotted line) and TOF-BPTV (black solid and dotted line) are presented in Fig. 6.37. It may be seen that the TOF-BPTV algorithm achieved slightly better PSF values in transverse direction (see Fig. 6.37 left panel), resulting in effective spatial resolution of $\sim 0.5 \div 0.8$ cm; PSF values provided by the TOF-FBP method are $\sim 0.7 \div 1.0$ cm. On the other hand, the estimated longitudinal resolution differs significantly for both methods (see Fig. 6.37 right panel). In this case, the TOF-BPTV algorithm provides almost twofold reduction in the PSF values compared to the TOF-FBP method.

In the last part of this study the computational speed of TOF-FBP and TOF-BPTV methods will be compared. For comparison purposes,

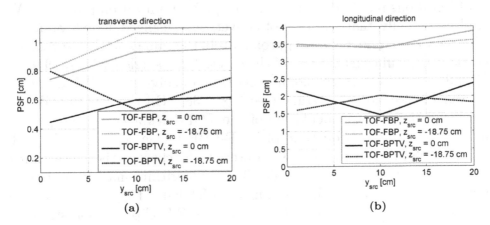

Figure 6.37. Estimated spatial resolution (FWHM) of the 3-layer prototype J-PET scanner calculated from experimental data, reconstructed by TOF-FBP and TOF-BPTV algorithms.

the number of coincident events from the experimental data considered during the reconstruction process was changed from 0.4 to 10.0 million. As in the previous studies with six point-like sources, the reconstruction volume was $50 \times 50 \times 50$ cm^3, comprising $125 \times 125 \times 125$ voxels. The results of comparative studies are summarized in Fig. 6.38. Note that the TOF-BPTV reconstruction encompasses two stages: calculation of TOF-backprojected image (see section 5.2.2 for details) and solving of the TV regularization problem (see section 5.2.3 for details). It should be stressed that the evaluation time of the latter stage is independent of the number of acquired coincident events (see black dotted line in Fig. 6.38 for details). The execution time of this stage depends on the overall num-

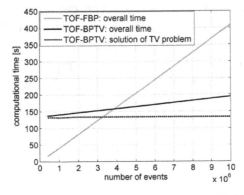

Figure 6.38. Comparison of the computational speed of TOF-FBP and TOF-BPTV methods using experimental data from the 3-layer J-PET detector.

ber of iterations required to solve the TV/L2 minimization problem. We found empirically that the rate of convergence using different values of regularization parameter μ is approximately the same and that seventeen iterations are sufficient in most of the cases. On a single CPU (Intel Core i5-5200U @ 2.20 GHz), the computing time of solving the TV/L2 problem was 133 seconds on average (see Fig. 6.38). On the other hand, the computing time of the calculation of the TOF-backprojected image and the overall reconstruction time of TOF-FBP image scale linearly with the number of considered events. However, the characteristic describing the computational speed of the TOF-FBP algorithm, marked with gray colour, is steeper than the line obtained for TOF-BPTV method, marked with black colour. The reason is that the TOF-backprojection stage relies exclusively on calculating the positions of the events in 3-D image space, the filtration using the operator a is performed during the latter stage. In contrast, the TOF-FBP algorithm applies three additional kernels, i.e., along LOR and its perpendicular direction and along axial direction, to each event [108]. From Fig. 6.38 it may be seen that the overall computing time is the same for both methods for about 3.9 million coincidence events. For a larger data set, the TOF-BPTV method is more computationally efficient than the TOF-FBP reconstruction. For instance, on the same CPU, the overall computing time for 10.0 million coincidence events was approximately 2.1 times shorter for TOF-BPTV method than required by TOF-FBP reconstruction, i.e., in the first case the time was 195 s and in the second case was 408 s on average.

It should be stressed that the computing time of the TOF-BPTV method strongly depends on the operator a size. During preliminary studies an investigation for the potential introduction of error due to truncation on different distances from the center of the kernel a along (x, y, z) directions, from 2.0σ to 4.0σ, was performed. Our tests revealed that 3.0σ seemed to be the optimal option for balance between quality degradation and acceleration of the reconstruction process. This value was used throughout the studies described in this work.

7. Conclusions and summary

The J-PET collaboration brings together scientists from different disciplines in order to develop a more affordable whole-body PET scanner. The application of the plastic scintillators entails the desing of unique detector geometry, dedicated electronics and reconstruction algorithms. Studies presented in this dissertation cover the analysis of the data processing in the J-PET scanner.

The operational principles of the J-PET scanner are similar to state-of-the-art PET detectors, except that the extremely precise time information is of paramount importance. In the J-PET, the time resolution influences not only the uncertainty of position reconstruction along the LOR, as in case of the conventional PET systems, but also has an impact on the uncertainty of position reconstruction along the scintillator strip. Therefore, the J-PET detector requires a development of novel methods at each step of data processing. The problem of data processing has been split into two separate parts in order to distinguish the low-level signal recovery and reconstruction from the high-level image processing. The goal of the low-level data processing is an evaluation of the information about each event of positron-electron annihilation based on the raw signals acquired during the PET examination. This information includes the estimated values of position and time of annihilation and deposited energy by two γ photons in the scintillators. In the next stage, denoted in this work as high-level data processing, the list of reconstructed events of positron-electron annihilations is subjected to further analysis with the primary goal of estimating the radioactive tracer distribution after injection into the patient's body. Main achievements related to both stages of data processing in the J-PET tomography are shortly summarized in the next two sections.

7.1 Summary of low-level data processing

In this dissertation a novel scheme of signal recovery in plastic scintillators in the J-PET scanner was introduced. The idea of signal recovery is based on the Tikhonov regularization theory, which uses the training data set of signals. The compact representation of these signals was provided by the PCA decomposition. One of the most important aspects of this part of research is the statistical analysis of the error level of recovered signals. The dependence of the signal recovery error on the number of samples taken in the voltage domain was determined and it has been proven that an average recovery error is approximately inversely proportional to the number of samples acquired in the voltage domain. It was shown that the PCA decomposition offers high levels of information compression and an accurate recovery may be provided with just eight samples for each signal waveform. It should be underlined that the developed recovery scheme is general and may be incorporated in any other investigation where prior knowledge about the signals of interest may be utilized.

In the experimental section, it was demonstrated that using the recovered signals improves the hit-position reconstruction. The experiments with the data set of signals from a single plastic scintillator strip show that the application of information from four voltage levels to the recovery of the signal waveform can improve the spatial resolution along the strip to about 0.94 cm. This result is about 0.1 cm better in comparison to the one estimated based on the eight samples per signal alone. It is worth noting that using more than four voltage levels does not provide significant improvements of spatial resolution. Future work will address development of more sophisticated methods to define the position and time of interaction of γ photon in the scintillator based on the recovered signal waveform. We believe that with fully recovered signals, there is still scope for improvement in the time and position resolution of the J-PET system.

Moreover, in this dissertation we introduced a new method for estimating the CRT of the J-PET detector. The basic idea of the prediction of time resolution is the use of the statistical nature of the acquisition process of the electric signals. The acqsution of the signals at the photomultipliers output is preceded by three main statistical phenomena: the emission of light photons in the scintillation material, the propagation of light pulses along the strip, and transition of the photoelectrons through the photomultiplier. One of the most important aspect of this part of work concerns the statistical analysis of a reconstruction error of the probability density function based on the set of single photoelectron signals. The dependences of the overall variance and bias on the number and width (standard deviation) of the single photoelectron signals were evaluated. The proposed estimation method was validated using the MC simulation and it was shown that the obtained results are consistent.

Furthermore, the developed estimation scheme was demonstrated to be
more accurate than the approach described in literature. It should be
stressed that the proposed method is general and may be incorporated
elsewhere.

It was demonstrated that the CRT obtained with the experimental
scheme with vacuum tube photomultipliers, reported to about 275 ps,
was very similar to the calculations with the proposed method which
results in time resolution of about 290 ps. The consistency of the experimental and theoretical results obtained for the J-PET detector equipped
with vacuum tube photomultipliers suggests that the estimated CRTs for
other photomultipliers are reliable. This aspect is of fundamental importance, as the accurate simulation tools are very useful for the design of
expensive devices such as the PET systems; in case of the J-PET scanner
the most expensive part of the system are the photomultipliers. Future
work will investigate other aspects of the signal acquisition process by
using the proposed statistical model, e.g., the influence of the parameters
describing the distribution of the photon emission time on the CRT. This
task is of main importance, since our group has developed a novel type of
plastic scintillator, similar to BC-420 used in this study, and provided the
examinations of the influence of the chemical composition of the plastic
scintillator on the overall performance of the J-PET system [110–112].

7.2   Summary of high-level data processing

In this dissertation a 3-dimensional image reconstruction algorithm dedicated for the TOF-PET scanners was introduced. The method takes
advantage of the TOF information, and the reconstruction problem is for-
mulated entirely in the image space, i.e., it includes TOF back-projected
data. This idea allowed us to convert the reconstruction problem of
the image to a regularization problem and, consequently, more advanced
techniques such as the TV method could be applied. In contrast to a
more traditional application of the TV regularization for PET data in
the projection space, the efficiency of our approach comes from the one-
time TOF back-projection step. The simulation study demonstrated that
the proposed reconstruction algorithm was faster than the TOF-FBP for
typical size of the data set with more than 4 million coincidence events.
Simultaneously, it was shown that the proposed method can perform
better in PET imaging than the TOF-MLEM algorithm.

The proposed approach requires the calculation of the kernel operator
$(a(\vec{x}))$ of the linear transform mapping an original radioactive tracer dis-

tribution into a TOF back-projected image. In this dissertation, it was shown that the function $a(\vec{x})$ may be approximated as the convolution of the three distributions describing the measurement imperfections: time measurement errors related to TOF resolution, non-zero size of the scintillator in (x, y) cross-section, and measurement errors along the strip. The operator $a(\vec{x})$ was derived for a spatially invariant system based on a point source placed in the center of the PET detector. Future work will address an incorporation of the shift variance technique in the image reconstruction process. Since the TV optimization in image space is very efficient it is advisable to incorporate the shift variance by evaluation of a set of operators $a(\vec{x}, \vec{x_p})$ for set of point sources $\vec{x_p}$ placed inside the detector volume. The operators $a(\vec{x}, \vec{x_p})$ may be simulated only for points $\vec{x_p}$ in 2-dimensional space, i.e., for point sources along the radial and axial directions, assuming that two points with the same axial and radial distance to the detector center share the same kernel $a(\vec{x}, \vec{x_p})$ after rotation in the transaxial plane. The regularization problem may be then modified so that for each operator $a(\vec{x}, \vec{x_p})$ a small sub-image centered at position $\vec{x_p}$ could be calculated independently. The final output image could be reconstructed as a weighted sum of the overlapping sub-images. This approach will require specifications of both spacing of the point sources $\vec{x_p}$ and percentage of the sub-images overlapping. This topic is related to existing work on non-stationary image PSF and on TOF spatial inhomogeneity [113] and will be investigated during further studies. We believe that the incorporation of the shift variance technique in the image reconstruction process will further improve the performance of the proposed method.

Appendix

A.1 Derivation of error resulting from signal recovery procedure

In the following we prove the theorem for average value of the recovery error (σ_x^2) introduced in section 4.2, in Eq. (4.20). We assume, for the sake of simplicity, that the matrix A, transforming the sparse expantion x into the signal y, has normally distributed elements with zero means and $1/N$ variances. These values of the parameters of normal distribution ensure that the matrix A is orthonormal. Hence, based on Eq. (4.17), the covariance matrix S_r is given by:

$$S_r = \left(P^{-1} + \sigma^2 \frac{M}{N} \mathbb{1} \right)^{-1} \tag{A.1}$$

where M is the number of acquired samples, N is the number of samples in complete signal, σ is standard deviation of noise in signal and P denotes the covariance matrix of a prior distribution of sparse expantion x. The σ_x^2 is equal to the trace of the matrix S_r and hence:

$$\begin{aligned}
\sigma_x^2 &= \sum_{k=1}^{N} \frac{\sigma^2 N P_{k,k}}{\sigma^2 N + M P_{k,k}} \\
&= \frac{\sigma^2 N^2}{M} \left(1 - \sigma^2 \sum_{k=1}^{N} \frac{1}{\sigma^2 N + M P_{k,k}} \right).
\end{aligned} \tag{A.2}$$

The sum in the last term in Eq. (A.2) may be approximated by a definite integral. In the following we will use for the calculations a basic rectangle rule, and:

$$\sum_{k=1}^{N} \frac{1}{\sigma^2 N + M P_{k,k}} \approx \int_{1-h}^{N+h} \frac{1}{\sigma^2 N + M P(k)} dk = \mathbf{I} \tag{A.3}$$

where $h = 1/2$. At the very beginning, see Eq. (4.19), we assumed that the function $P(k)$ has the form:

$$P(k) = D \cdot e^{-\tau k}. \tag{A.4}$$

We will perform the integration using the substitution $t = e^{-\tau k}$. Without any significant loss of precision, we change the integration limits from $[1 - h, \; N + h]$ to $[0, \; N]$. The calculations of the integral $\mathbf{I}$ will be as follows:

$$\mathbf{I} = \int_{e^{-\tau N}}^{1} \frac{1}{(\sigma^2 N + M D t)\, \tau t} dt$$

$$= \int_{e^{-\tau N}}^{1} \frac{1}{\sigma^2 N \tau t} dt - \int_{e^{-\tau N}}^{1} \frac{MD}{\sigma^2 N \tau (\sigma^2 N + M D t)} dt$$

$$= \frac{1}{\sigma^2 N \tau} \left(\log(t)\big|_{e^{-\tau N}}^{1} - \log(\sigma^2 N + M D t)\big|_{e^{-\tau N}}^{1} \right)$$

$$\approx \frac{1}{\sigma^2 N \tau} \left(N\tau + \log\left(\frac{\sigma^2 N}{\sigma^2 N + MD} \right) \right). \tag{A.5}$$

Finally, substituting the integral $\mathbf{I}$ in Eq. (A.5) into formula in Eq. (A.2), gives the average value of the recovery error:

$$\sigma_x^2 \approx \frac{\sigma^2 N^2}{M} \left(1 - \sigma^2 \mathbf{I} \right)$$

$$\approx \frac{\sigma^2 N}{M\tau} \cdot \log\left(\frac{\sigma^2 N + MD}{\sigma^2 N} \right).$$

A.2   Derivation of error resulting from limited number of photoelectrons

As mentioned in section 4.4.1, the function $\tilde{y}_k$, describing the kth signal from a single photoelectron is assumed to be a Gaussian function with standard deviation σ_p. The function $\tilde{y}_k$, given in Eq. (4.37), may be approximated with:

$$\tilde{y}_k(n) \approx \begin{cases} \frac{\beta}{\sqrt{(2\pi)N_p \sigma_p}} \left(1 - \frac{(t^{(n)} - t_r^k)^2}{\lambda^2 \sigma_p^2} \right) & t_r^k \in (t^{(n)} - \lambda\sigma_p, t^{(n)} + \lambda\sigma_p) \\ 0 & \text{otherwise} \end{cases}$$

$$\tag{A.6}$$

where t_r^k is a random variable with f_{t_r} distribution, which denotes the kth photon's registration time, λ contributes to the signal width and $n = 1, 2, ..., N$. The probability that the random variable $\tilde{y}_k(n)$ is equal to the specified value may be calculated based on the previously introduced function Φ

$$\Phi(t^{(n)}, \lambda\sigma_p) = F_{t_r}(t^{(n)} + \lambda\sigma_p) - F_{t_r}(t^{(n)} - \lambda\sigma_p), \qquad n = 1, 2, ..., N,$$

see Eq. (4.46). In particular, the probability that the random variable $\tilde{y}_k(n) = 0$ is equal to $1 - \Phi(t^{(n)}, \lambda\sigma_p)$; the kth registration time t_r^k is out of range $(t^{(n)} - \lambda\sigma_p, t^{(n)} + \lambda\sigma_p)$, see the second case in Eq. (A.6). Denoting the first case in Eq. (A.6) with u_k :

$$u_k(n) = \frac{\beta}{\sqrt{(2\pi)}N_p\sigma_p} \left(1 - \frac{(t^{(n)} - t_r^k)^2}{\lambda^2\sigma_p^2} \right), \quad n = 1, 2, ..., N, \quad (A.7)$$

we may write that for $n = 1, 2, ..., N$, the expected value of $\tilde{y}_k(n)$ is equal:

$$E[\tilde{y}_k(n)] = E[u_k(n)]\Phi(t^{(n)}, \lambda\sigma_p) + E[0](1 - \Phi(t^{(n)}, \lambda\sigma_p))$$
$$= E[u_k(n)]\Phi(t^{(n)}, \lambda\sigma_p), \quad (A.8)$$

and the variance of $\tilde{y}_k(n)$ is equal:

$$\mathrm{Var}(\tilde{y}_k(n)) = E[(u_k(n) - E[u_k(n)])^2]\Phi(t^{(n)}, \lambda\sigma_p) +$$
$$E[(0 - E[u_k(n)])^2](1 - \Phi(t^{(n)}, \lambda\sigma_p))$$
$$= \mathrm{Var}(\tilde{u}_k(n))\Phi(t^{(n)}, \lambda\sigma_p) + E[u_k(n)]^2(1 - \Phi(t^{(n)}, \lambda\sigma_p)).$$
$$(A.9)$$

In order to simplify the further calculations the following assumption is proposed. Note that in most interesting cases the range $(t^{(n)} - \lambda\sigma_p, t^{(n)} + \lambda\sigma_p)$, is narrow in comparison to the estimated pdf function f_{t_r} domain. Therefore, the pdf function f_{t_r} is considered to be uniform in the range $(t^{(n)} - \lambda\sigma_p, t^{(n)} + \lambda\sigma_p)$:

$$f_{t_r}(\epsilon) \simeq \text{const.} \quad \epsilon \in (t^{(n)} - \lambda\sigma_p, t^{(n)} + \lambda\sigma_p). \quad (A.10)$$

It is worth noting that the smaller the ratio of the single to overall signal width is, the better is the performance of the proposed approximation method.

Under the assumption in Eq. (A.10), required moments in Eqs. (A.8) and (A.9), $E[u_k(n)]$, $E[u_k(n)]^2$ and $\mathrm{Var}(\tilde{u}_k(n))$, can be easily derived. After some simple calculations the equations for the expected value and the variance of the random variable $\tilde{y}_k(n)$ are given by formulas[1]:

$$E(\tilde{y}(n)) \approx \beta\frac{2\Phi(t^{(n)}, \lambda\sigma_p)}{3\sqrt{2\pi}\sigma_p},$$

$$\mathrm{Var}(\tilde{y}(n)) \approx \beta^2\frac{9\Phi(t^{(n)}, \lambda\sigma_p) + 8\Phi^2(t^{(n)}, \lambda\sigma_p) - 16\Phi^3(t^{(n)}, \lambda\sigma_p)}{36\pi N_p\sigma_p^2},$$

for $n = 1, 2, ..., N$.

[1] L. Raczyński et al., Calculation of the time resolution of the J-PET tomograph using kernel density estimation, *Phys. Med. Biol.* **62** (2017) 5095.

A.3   Derivation of convolution operator a

In the following we will show a derivation of pdfs $a_{(1)}, a_{(2)}, a_{(3)}$ describing the operator a mapping an original radioactive tracer distribution into a TOF back-projected image.

The proposed image reconstruction method was introduced in section 5.2. The functions $a_{(1)}, a_{(2)}, a_{(3)}$ describe the pds of measurement errors $\vec{\epsilon_1}, \vec{\epsilon_2}, \vec{\epsilon_3}$, respectively. In most cases it is convenient to model the error distributions in projection space, and $p_{(k)}^\delta$ describes the pdf of projection data of a point source $\delta(\vec{x})$ affected with errors introduced only by k^{th} components in Eq. (5.20).

A.3.1   Calculation of operator $a_{(1)}$

As described in section 5.2.2 we assume that the $\vec{\epsilon_1}$ depends only on time uncertainties $(t_{u,e}, t_{d,e})$. Therefore, the pdf of projection data $p_{(1)}^\delta$ considers only the TOF variable and according to Eq. (5.8):

$$p_{(1)}^\delta(\vec{\Sigma}) = \int_{-\infty}^{\infty} dl' \delta(\vec{x} = l'\vec{\omega_1})h(l - l') = h(l\vec{\omega_1}) \qquad (A.11)$$

where function h describes the TOF profile. The back-projection of the projection data $p_{(1)}^\delta$ onto the image space is given as:

$$a_{(1)}(\vec{x}) = (\mathcal{K}^\# p_{(1)}^\delta)(\vec{x}) = \int_0^{\theta_{acc}} d\theta \int_0^\pi d\phi \int_{-\infty}^{\infty} dl h(l\vec{\omega_1}). \qquad (A.12)$$

It is convenient to convert the spherical coordinates in the above integral to Cartesian coordinates $\vec{u} = (u, v, w)$. The equations to convert between Cartesian and spherical coordinates are:

$$l = \sqrt{u^2 + v^2 + w^2}$$

$$\phi = \arctan\left(\frac{u}{v}\right)$$

$$\theta = \arccos\left(\frac{w}{\sqrt{u^2 + v^2 + w^2}}\right).$$

The transformation between coordinate systems is given by:

$$dl d\phi d\theta = \begin{vmatrix} \frac{dl}{du} & \frac{dl}{dv} & \frac{dl}{dw} \\ \frac{d\phi}{du} & \frac{d\phi}{dv} & \frac{d\phi}{dw} \\ \frac{d\theta}{du} & \frac{d\theta}{dv} & \frac{d\theta}{dw} \end{vmatrix} du dv dw = \frac{d\vec{u}}{\|\vec{u}\|\sqrt{u^2 + v^2}}$$

and finally:

$$a_{(1)}(\vec{x}) = \kappa_1 \frac{h(\|\vec{x}\|)\mathcal{C}(\vec{x}, \theta_{\text{acc}})}{\|\vec{x}\|\sqrt{x^2 + y^2}}$$

where κ_1 stands for the normalization constant and the function $\mathcal{C}(\vec{x}, \theta_{\text{acc}})$ is defined as:

$$\mathcal{C}(\vec{x}, \theta_{\text{acc}}) = \begin{cases} 1 & \frac{z}{\|\vec{x}\|} \leq \cos\theta_{\text{acc}} \\ 0 & \text{otherwise.} \end{cases} \tag{A.13}$$

The function $\mathcal{C}(\vec{x}, \theta_{\text{acc}})$ originates from the integration limit θ_{acc} of the θ angle in Eq. (A.12).

A.3.2   Calculation of operator $a_{(2)}$

As described in section 5.2.2 the $\vec{\epsilon_2}$ depends only on transaxial uncertainties $(x_{u,e}, y_{u,e}, x_{d,e}, y_{d,e})$. Therefore, the pdf of projection data $p_{(2)}^\delta$ may be described as:

$$p_{(2)}^\delta(\vec{\Sigma}) = \int_{-\infty}^{\infty} dl'\delta(\vec{x} = l'\vec{\omega_2^\perp})h_2(l - l') = h_2(l\vec{\omega_2^\perp}) \tag{A.14}$$

where the profile function $h_2(l)$ has a triangle distribution:

$$h_2(l) = \begin{cases} \frac{2D - 4|l|}{D^2} & |l| \leq \frac{D}{2} \\ 0 & \text{otherwise} \end{cases} \tag{A.15}$$

where D is the thickness of the plastic scintillator. The function $h_2(l)$ originates from the fact that the depth of interaction is unknown and we assume the midpoint of the strip as the measured position in (x, y) cross-section (see estimates $x_{d,e}, x_{u,e}$ in Fig. 5.2).

The back-projection of the projection data $p_{(2)}^\delta$ onto the image space is given as:

$$a_{(2)}(\vec{x}) = (\mathcal{K}^\# p_{(2)}^\delta)(\vec{x}) = \int_0^{\theta_{\text{acc}}} d\theta \int_0^\pi d\phi \int_{-\infty}^\infty dl h_2(l\vec{\omega_2^\perp})$$

$$= \int_0^\pi d\phi \int_{-\infty}^\infty dl h_2(l\vec{\omega_2^\perp}) \tag{A.16}$$

and does not depend on the θ angle. It is convenient to convert the polar coordinates in the above integral to Cartesian coordinates. The equations to convert between Cartesian and polar coordinates are:

$$l = \sqrt{u^2 + v^2}$$

$$\phi = \arctan\left(\frac{u}{v}\right).$$

The transformation between coordinate systems is:

$$dl\,d\phi = \begin{vmatrix} \frac{dl}{du} & \frac{dl}{dv} \\ \frac{d\phi}{du} & \frac{d\phi}{dv} \end{vmatrix} du\,dv = \frac{du\,dv}{\sqrt{u^2 + v^2}}$$

and finally:

$$a_{(2)}(\vec{x}) = \kappa_2 \frac{h_2(\sqrt{x^2 + y^2})}{\sqrt{x^2 + y^2}}$$

where κ_2 stands for the normalization constant.

A.3.3   Calculation of operator $a_{(3)}$

As described in section 5.2.2 the $\vec{\epsilon_3}$ depends only on axial uncertainties $(z_{u,e}, z_{d,e})$. In this case the calculations do not involve the analysis of pdf of errors in projection space. Note that:

$$\vec{\epsilon_3} = \frac{z_{d,e} + z_{u,e}}{2} \tag{A.17}$$

and under the assumption that the uncertainty of the measurement of axial positions $z_{u,e}, z_{d,e}$ are a Gaussian function with standard deviation σ_z that does not depend on the position along the strip, the pdf $a_{(3)}$ is given as:

$$a_{(3)}(\vec{x}) = \frac{1}{\sqrt{\pi}\sigma_z} \exp\left(-\frac{z}{\sigma_z^2}\right). \tag{A.18}$$

References

[1] L. Raczyński et al., *Nucl. Instr. & Meth.* **A 764** (2014) 168.

[2] L. Raczyński et al., *Nucl. Instr. & Meth.* **A 786** (2015) 105.

[3] L. Raczyński et al., *Nukleonika* **61** (2016) 35.

[4] L. Raczyński et al., *Phys. Med. Biol.* **62** (2017) 5076.

[5] L. Raczyński et al., *Acta Phys. Pol.* **B 48** (2017) 1611.

[6] L. Raczyński et al., *Acta Phys. Pol.* **B 51** (2020) 175.

[7] L. Raczyński et al., *Phys. Med.: Eur. J. Med. Phys.* **80** (2020) 230.

[8] J. L. Humm et al., *European J. of Nucl. Med. & Mol. Imag.* **30** (2003) 1574.

[9] D. L. Bailey, *Positron Emission Tomography: Basic Sciences*, Springer-Verlag, New York (2005).

[10] H. H. Barrett, T. White, L. C. Parra, *J. Amer. Stat. Assoc.* **14** (1997) 2914.

[11] P. Słomka, T. Pan, G. Germano, *Semin. Nucl. Med.* **46** (2016) 5.

[12] J. van Sluis et al., *J. Nucl. Med.* **60** (2019) 1031.

[13] T. Budinger, *J. Nucl. Med.* **24** (1983) 73.

[14] S. Seifert S, H. T. van Dam, D. R. Schaart, *Phys. Med. Biol.* **57** (2012) 1797.

[15] D. R. Schaart, S. Seifert, R. Vinke, H. T. van Dam, P. Dendooven, H. Lohner, F. J. Beekman, *Phys. Med. Biol.* **55** (2010) N179.

[16] P. Lecoq, *IEEE Trans. Radiat. Plasma Med. Sci.* **1** (2017) 473.

[17] P. Moskal et al., *Nucl. Instr. & Meth.* **A 764** (2014) 317.

[18] P. Moskal et al., *Nucl. Instr. & Meth.* **A 775** (2015) 54.

[19] P. Moskal et al., *Phys. Med. Biol.* **61** (2016) 2025.

[20] S. Niedźwiecki et al., *Acta Phys. Pol.* **B 48** (2017) 1567.

[21] M. Gierlik et al., *Nucl. Instr. & Meth.* **A 593** (2008) 426.

[22] S. Ashrafi, M. G. Gol, *Nucl. Instr. & Meth.* **A 642** (2011) 70.

[23] G. L. Brownell, C. A. Burnham, B. Hoop Jr, D. E. Bohning (eds.), Dynamic Studies with Radioisotopes in Medicine. Proceedings of the Symposium on Dynamics Studies with Radioisotopes in Clinical Medicine and Research, Rotterdam (1970), Int. Atomic Energy Agency, Vienna (1971).

[24] J. S. Robertson et al., *Tomo. Imag. Nucl. Med.* (1973) 142.

[25] Z. H. Cho, L. Eriksson, J. K. Chan, *Int. J. Nucl. Med. Biol.* **3** (1976) 165.

[26] T. Ido, C. N. Wan, V. Casella, J. S. Fowler, A. P. Wolf, M. Reivich, D. E. Kuhl, *J. Labelled Comp. Radiopharm.* **14** (1978) 175.

[27] A. S. Crespo, P. Andreo, S. A. Larsson, *European J. of Nucl. Med. & Mol. Imag.* **31** (2004) 44.

[28] G. F. Knoll, *Radiation Detection and Measurement*, John Wiley & Sons, New York (2000).

[29] G. B. Saha, *Basics of PET Imaging: Physics, Chemistry, and Regulations*, Springer, New York (2005).

[30] K. Szymański et al., *Bio-Algorithms Med. Syst.* **10** (2014) 71.

[31] J. H. Hubbell, *Phys. Med. Biol.* **44** (1999) R1.

[32] Saint Gobain Crystals 2016 http://www.crystals.saint-gobain.com.

[33] M. Conti, *Phys. Med.* **25** (2009) 1.

[34] Hamamatsu Handbook, *Photomultiplier Tubes Basics and Applications, Hamamatsu Photonics*, Electron Tube Division (2007).

[35] P. E. Valk, D. L. Bailey, D. W. Townsend, M. N. Maisey, *Positron Emission Tomography: Basic Science and Clinical Practice*, Springer (2003).

[36] M. E. Casey, R. Nutt, *IEEE Trans. Nucl. Sci.* **NS-33** (1986) 460.

[37] S. R. Cherry, *J. Nucl. Med.* **47** (2006) 1735.

[38] S. Vandenberghe et al., *EJNMMI Physics* **3** (2016) 1.

[39] N. A. Karakatsanis, M. A. Lodge, A. K. Tahari, Y. Zhou, R. L. Wahl, A. Rahmim, *Phys. Med. Biol.* **58** (2013) 7391.

[40] X. Zhang, J. Zhou, G. Wang, J. K. Poon, S. R. Cherry, R. D. Badawi, J Qi, *J. Nucl. Med.* **55** (2014) 269.

[41] S. R. Cherry, R. D. Badawi, J. S. Karp, W. W. Moses, P. Price, T. Jones, *Sci. Trans. Med.* **9** (2017) 381.

[42] R. D. Badawi et al., *J. Nucl. Med.* **60** (2019) 299.

[43] X. Zhang X et al., *Phys. Med. Biol.* **62** (2017) 2465.

[44] A. Strzelecki, PhD thesis, Dept. Polish Acad. Sci., Institute Fundamental Technological Research, Kraków (2016).

[45] G. Korcyl et al., *Acta Phys. Pol.* **B 47** (2016) 491.

[46] J. Smyrski et al., *Nucl. Instr. & Meth.* **A 851** (2017) 39.

[47] M. Traxler et al., *J. Instrum.* **6** (2011) C12004.

[48] C. Ugur, G. Korcyl, J. Michel, M. Penschuk, M. Traxler, *Proceedings of the IEEE Nordic-Medit.* Workshop Time-Digit (2013).

[49] G. Korcyl, PhD thesis, Univ. Science Technology, Kraków (2015).

[50] G. Korcyl et al., *IEEE Trans. Med. Imag.* **37** (2018) 2526.

[51] M. Pałka et al., *J. Instrum.* **12** (2017) P08001.

[52] E. Candes, J. Romberg, T. Tao, *IEEE Trans. Information Theory* **52** (2006) 489.

[53] D. Donoho, *IEEE Trans. Information Theory* **52** (2006) 1289.

[54] S. Mallat, Z. Zhang, *IEEE Trans. Sig. Proc.* **41** (1993) 3397.

[55] S. Chen, D. Donoho, M. Saunders, *SIAM J. Scien. Comp.* **20** (1998) 33.

[56] E. Candes, T. Tao, *IEEE Trans. Information Theory* **51** (2005) 4203.

[57] E. Candes, J. Romberg, T. Tao, *Comm. Pure Appl. Math.* **59** (2006) 1207.

[58] L. I. Rudin, S. Osher, E. Fatemi, *Physica D* **60** (1992) 259.

[59] G. Golub, C. van Loan, *Matrix Computation*, MD: Johns Hopkins Univ. Press, Baltimore (1989).

[60] Y. Huang, M. K. Ng, Y. Wen, *SIAM Multisc. Model Simul.* **7** (2008) 774.

[61] S. H. Chan, R. Khoshabeh, K. B. Gibson, P. E. Gill, T. Q. Nguyen, *IEEE Trans. Imag. Process.* **20** (2011) 3097.

[62] M. Elad, *IEEE Trans. Information Theory* **52** (2006) 5559.

[63] T. Kohonen, *Self-Organizing Maps*, Springer, Berlin (1995).

[64] Q. Xie et al., *IEEE Trans. Nucl. Sci.* **NS-56** (2009) 2607.

[65] H. Kim et al., *Nucl. Instr. & Meth.* **A 602** (2009) 618.

[66] M. Moszynski, B. Bengtson, *Nucl. Instr. & Meth.* **A 142** (1977) 417.

[67] M. Moszynski, B. Bengtson, *Nucl. Instr. & Meth.* **A 158** (1979) 1.

[68] A. Tikhonov, *Soviet Math. Dokl.* 4 (1963) 1035.

[69] A. Tikhonov, V. Arsenin, *Solutions of Ill-Posed Problems*, Winston and Sons, Washington, D.C. (1977).

[70] D. P. Berrar et al., *A Practical Approach to Microarray Data Analysis*, Kluwer Academic Publishers, Boston (2002).

[71] P. Hansen, *Rank-Deficient and Discrete Ill-Posed Problems. Numerical Aspects of Linear Inversion*, SIAM, Philadelphia (1997).

[72] R. Kalman, *Trans. ASME - J. Basic Eng.* (1960) 35.

[73] H. Sorenson, *IEEE Spectrum* **7** (1970) 63.

[74] K. V. Mardia, *Biometrika* **57** (1970) 519.

[75] H. W. Lilliefors, *J. Am. Stat. Assoc.* **62** (1967) 399.

[76] L. Fattorini, *Statistica* **2** (1986) 209.

[77] J. Villasenor Alva, E. González Estrada, *Comm. Stat. Theory Methods* **38** (2009) 1870.

[78] M. B. Wilk, R. Gnanadesikan, *Biometrika* **55** (1968) 1.

[79] R. A. Johnson et al. (eds.) *Applied Multivariate Statistical Analysis*, Prentice Hall, New Jersey (1992)

[80] T. Bednarski et al., *Bio-Algorithms Med. Syst.* **10** (2014) 13.

[81] M. Rosenblat, *Ann. Math. Stat.* **27** (1956) 832.

[82] J. Simonoff, *Smoothing Methods in Statistics*, Springer, New York (1996).

[83] A. Rahmim, M. Lenox, A. J. Reader, C. Michel, Z. Burbar, T. J. Ruth, V. Sossi, *Phys. Med. Biol.* **49** (2004) 4239.

[84] R. Accorsi, L. E. Adam, M. E. Werner, J. S. Karp, *Phys. Med. Biol.* **49** (2004) 2577.

[85] C. C. Watson, *IEEE Trans. Nucl. Sci.* **54** (2007) 1679.

[86] R. M. Gray, *IEEE ASSP Magazine* **1** (1984) 4.

[87] H. Jegou, M. Douze, C. Schmid, *IEEE Trans. Pattern Anal. Machine Intelligence* **33** (2011) 117.

[88] V. Westerwoudt, M. Conti, L. Eriksson, *IEEE Trans. Nucl. Sci.* **61** (2014) 126.

[89] R. Bates, T. Peters, *New Zealand Jour. Sci.* **14** (1971) 883.

[90] M. Defrise, M. E. Casey, C. Michel, M. Conti, *Phys. Med. Biol.* **50** (2005) 2749.

[91] Y. Li, S. Matej, S. D. Metzler, *Phys. Med. Biol.* **61** (2016) 601.

[92] M. Conti, B. Bendriem, M. Casey, M. Chen, F. Kehren, C. Michel, V. Panin, *Phys. Med. Biol.* **50** (2005) 4507.

[93] D. L. Snyder, L. J. Thomas, M. M. Ter-Pogossian, *IEEE Trans. Nucl. Sci.* (1982) 3575.

[94] A. Mallon, P. Grangeat, *Phys. Med. Biol.* **37** (1992) 717.

[95] Z. H. Cho, J. B. Ra, S. K. Hilal, *IEEE Trans. Med. Imag.* **1** (1983) 6.

[96] P. E. Kinahan, J. G. Rogers, *IEEE Trans. Nucl. Sci.* **36** (1989) 964.

[97] P. E. Barbano, A. Fokas, C. Schonlieb, *Proceedings of the International Conf. Sampta Singapore* (2011).

[98] M. Burger, J. Muller, E. Papoutsellis, C. B. Schonlieb, *Inv. Probl.* **30** (2014) 105003.

[99] L. A. Shepp, Y. Vardi, *IEEE Trans. Med. Imag.* **1** (1982) 113.

[100] L. A. Shepp, Y. Vardi, *J. Amer. Stat. Assoc.* **2** (1985) 389.

[101] NEMA Standards Publication NU 2-2012: Performance measurements of Positron Emission Tomographs, Nat. Elect. Manuf. Assoc., Washington, D.C. (2012).

[102] P. Kowalski et al., *Acta Phys. Pol.* **B 47** (2016) 549.

[103] S. Jan et al., *Phys. Med. Biol.* **49** (2004) 4543.

[104] S. Jan et al., *Phys. Med. Biol.* **56** (2011) 881.

[105] E. Parzen, *Ann. Math. Stat.* **33** (1962) 1065.

[106] R. A. Fisher, *Annals of Eugenics* **7** (1936) 179.

[107] T. Merlin, S. Stute, D. Benoit, J. Bert, T. Carlier, C. Comtat, M. Filipovic, F. Lamare, D. Visvikis, *Phys. Med. Biol.* **63** (2018) 5505.

[108] R. Y. Shopa, *Acta Phys. Pol.* **B 51** (2020) 181.

[109] T. Tomitani, *IEEE Trans. Nucl. Sci.* **8** (1981) 4582.

[110] A. Wieczorek et al., *Nukleonika* **60** (2015) 777.

[111] A. Wieczorek et al., *Acta Phys. Pol.* **A 127** (2015) 1487.

[112] A. Wieczorek et al., *PLoS ONE* **12** (2017) 186728.

[113] E. Clementel, P. Mollet, S. Vandenberghe, *IEEE Trans. Nucl. Sci.* **60** (2013) 1578.

COPY EDITOR
Rafał Pawluk

TYPESETTER
Lech Raczyński

Jagiellonian University Press
Editorial Offices: Michałowskiego 9/2, 31-126 Kraków
Phone: +48 12 663 23 80, Fax: +48 12 663 23 83

CPSIA information can be obtained
at www.ICGtesting.com
Printed in the USA
JSHW051502140323
38869JS00010B/103